The Healthcare Assembly

Status One

Samuel Forman
Matthew Kelliher

Status One

. . . .

Breakthroughs in High Risk
Population Health Management

Jossey-Bass Publishers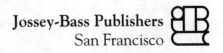
San Francisco

Jossey-Bass books and products are available through most bookstores. To contact Jossey-Bass directly, call (888) 378-2537, fax to (800) 605-2665, or visit our website at www.josseybass.com.

Substantial discounts on bulk quantities of Jossey-Bass books are available to corporations, professional associations, and other organizations. For details and discount information, contact the special sales department at Jossey-Bass.

 Manufactured in the United States of America on Lyons Falls Turin Book. This paper is acid-free and 100 percent totally chlorine-free.

Library of Congress Cataloging-in-Publication Data

Forman, Samuel.
    Status one : breakthroughs in high risk population health management / Samuel Forman and Matthew Kelliher.
        p. cm.
    Includes bibliographical references and index.
    ISBN 0-7879-4154-9 (hc : alk. paper)
    1. Managed care plans (Medical care)—Patients—Care.
2. Patients—Care—Quality control.   3. Medical care—Needs
assessment.   4. Health services accessibility.   I. Kelliher, Matthew.
II. Title.
RA413.F59   1999   99-18725
362.1–DC21   CIP

FIRST EDITION
HB Printing   10 9 8 7 6 5 4 3 2 1

Contents

*Part Three: Alternate Approaches to
    Medical Management*

Part Four: Sources and Rationale

Part Five: Putting It Together

Preface

. . . .

The Status One patient is at great risk in the near term for their own quality of life and presents a significant risk to the financial performance of their health care organization.

As managed care grows nationally and financial risk is shifted to provider groups, the need to truly redesign clinical care and improve its quality has never been greater. The contractual arrangements, fee discounting, and utilization barriers trumpeted as managed care since the late 1980s have proven inadequate. Solutions are much less apparent than the problem.

Clinicians and health care leaders have long recognized that a small subset of patients accounts for a disproportionate share of medical cost. In the absence of practical methods to proactively identify these patients and optimize their care, and with conflicting financial incentives to provide repeated episodes of care, this segment has been a neglected but costly group caught within the managed care system. So neglected are they, in fact, that as a group they have neither a name nor broad-based recognition of their impact on managed care. We refer to this group of patients as Status One.

The name *Status One* was chosen for this group because it conveys both clinical and economic urgency. Innovative health professionals are enthusiastically taking the Status One name and concepts to heart. They know and have lived the health experience of what is called Code Blue or Code 99: the immediacy of cardiopulmonary arrest and the variety of life-saving interventions for it. They also know about ambulatory and inpatient care and their implications. Status One gives a name to what physicians, nurses, and administrators instinctively know: there is a class of patients whose unique and complex needs are poorly met and whose costs of care are burdensome in a managed care environment.

This book is intended to help leaders in health care and managed care focus their organizations' competencies and priorities on the most vulnerable patients. If we cannot get care right for the Status One patient, how can we take any consolation in the "gains" made in improving quality in the health care system? Every friend or family member who has ever had to facilitate care of a Status One patient close to them understands the problems and the challenges we face. By virtue of their clinical instability and financial impact, Status One patients invite initiatives to improve their care. Such efforts complement more familiar clinical initiatives aimed at specific conditions—disease management.

This book outlines the challenges and opportunities. It begins with an overview in Chapter One, where we explain the current and future role of high-risk population health management.

Part Two describes the main components of a population health management strategy. Chapter Two describes ways of stratifying a population according to future risk of high costs and clinical complexity. Chapter Three addresses the use of information systems and the internet as a means to integrate the new approach to high-risk patient care. Chapter Four suggests ways to adapt current clinical organizations so that they can care for their Status One patients.

Chapters Five, Six, and Seven explore practical approaches to integrating patient priorities, providing psychosocial and medical care, meeting the needs of patients, formulating care plans, and reassessing and discharging patients. Included are the six aims for managing high-risk patients. Chapter Eight discusses essential process and outcome measures.

Sharply focused medical management for these medically needy and unstable patients contrasts with current practices. The next few chapters describe alternative approaches to medical management. Chapter Nine surveys the variety of methodologies that have traditionally been employed to identify clinically needy or costly patients. Chapters Ten and Eleven compare and contrast proactive, high-risk ambulatory-care management to more traditional case management and disease management programs. Chapter Twelve discusses intriguing new directions that become available when we segment patients according to future economic risk.

The sources and rationale that form the foundation of high-risk population health management are discussed in the final chapters. Tenets of quality management that can be applied to high-risk population health management are the subject of Chapter Thirteen. Epidemiological concepts and interpretations of their application to the structure and economics of the health care industry are the subject of Chapters Fourteen and Fifteen.

Chapter Sixteen is a summary of the approach to high-risk population health management.

Throughout the book we supply clinical anecdotes and case examples that illustrate key points. The cases are real. We have changed the names, altered demographics, and condensed them so that they preserve the confidentiality of the individuals and their families.

In the long term the health care delivery system could, on humanitarian grounds, apply high-risk population health management to all communities, regardless of size or location. In the current capitated environment, population health management is a critical managed care strategy for those bearing financial risk for health services.

This book is the first of its kind in the emerging and specialized field of population health management, which is critical to the future of managed care. HMOs have long aspired to coordinate care, improve quality, and demonstrate cost effectiveness. Medical management that delivers on these promises has yet to become the norm. We hope that the concepts presented in this book will stimulate a critical reexamination of and improvement in how the sickest people are treated.

Managed care organizations face one challenge above all others: lowering the cost of care while at the same time refining and improving the quality of that care. Interestingly, this individualized approach also improves the functional status, self-reliance, and productivity of those most burdened with illness. Leaders can meet this challenge head-on by adopting a population-oriented view of their delivery systems and directing initial efforts to managing that small group of needy people now.

Those organizations meeting this challenge will thrive in the future as managed care continues to expand into the dominant form of health care in the United States. Those organizations that simply focus on reducing costs by implementing cost-cutting measures that hurt patients and that ignore the requirement to increase quality will fail. The challenge is Status One, indeed!

Hopkinton, Massachusetts   Samuel Forman
April 1999   Matthew Kelliher

Acknowledgments

To Status One patients, among whom we might easily find our family members and friends, we dedicate this book. It is our modest attempt to redirect modern managed care to meet their needs rather than to let them fend for themselves in an often fragmented and, at best, reactive health care system.

Describing a new strategy poses some challenges for both authors and the reader. We want to acknowledge them now, in the spirit of being straightforward about the strengths and limitations of the material that follows. Many of what we identify as best practices are so contemporary that critical descriptions in the peer-reviewed scientific literature are rare. In the course of our interactions with a variety of managed care organizations, and the physicians, nurses, social workers, and administrators who enliven them, we have encountered and often incorporated into our own practice innovations that meet the criteria of raising functional health while reducing medical costs in the short term. We identify such practices as based on our experience. We cite medical and managed care trade journals on occasion but admonish the reader that such articles are based on other people's opinions and would pass hurdles neither of the double-blind, randomized clinical trial sort nor of peer review. We cite scientific literature when it exists.

We are indebted to Sanford Kurtz and Sam Nussbaum, early innovators and leaders, along with their organizations, of high-risk population health management.

For the concept of and lessons learned in managing high-risk patients we gratefully acknowledge social workers Marianne LoGerfo and Suzy Favaro of the North Shore Senior Center of Seattle/King County. Their programs and teaching have opened our eyes to the possibilities of fusing the fulfillment of psychological and social needs into a more traditional clinical model of patient care.

For insight, leadership, and foresight in organizations that have been early adopters of these concepts, we wish to recognize and thank John Lynch, Mark Gunby, Sandy Graff and Pierre Moeser of the BJC Health System in Missouri, and Jerry Maliot, Rob Schreiber, and Steve Moskowitz of the Lahey Clinic in eastern Massachusetts. As leading innovators and practitioners of Status One care management, we recognize Debbie Feldman, Vicki Morgan, Judy Ehrlich, Marianne Clark, Maxine Johnson, Pam Townsend, Sharon Johnson, Sharon Matthews, Sylvia Sanderson, and Lei Woods-Neal of Health Management Partners of Missouri.

For work on the conceptual predecessor program at the former delivery system at Blue Cross/Blue Shield of Massachusetts, we acknowledge the medical leadership, quality improvement staff, home care, and care coordinators—among them John Collins, Jonathan Forman, Helen Hendricks, Cathy Kowal, Jane Brazeau, Christina Phillipi, Joanne Bloom, and Ginny Burke.

We are indebted to Bill Wellman of First Consulting Group for insights on conceptualizing data needs and communications, observations that we incorporated into Chapter Three. Paul Coggin of Merck-MedCo educated us on the resources and initiatives of pharmaceutical benefit managers.

Colleagues at StatusOne Health Systems contributed immeasurably with their ideas and experience. Susan Neckes shared her experience with and insights into project initiation, resources, staffing, and training in building case management to effectively serve the highest-risk patients, as well as providing a critical reading of the book manuscript. Gary Wood contributed an understanding of the practical aspects of clinical information systems and the internet. Don Williams performed several of the analyses involving alternate approaches to high-risk patient identification.

To the leaders and staff of the Healthcare Assembly, thank you for your support and direction.

To delightful daughters, Rachel and Jennifer Forman, I extend my thanks and hugs for their forbearance while their daddy spent too many weekends writing and revising. To Pat, Brennan Marie, and Tory Kelliher, I extend thanks for the encouragement to go forward on the strength of my convictions. To Matt Senior and Ann Kelliher, I thank you for years and years of encouragement.

We encourage the many leaders, physicians, and nurses associated with managed care to rethink and to constantly improve the care for frail and acutely ill patients. These individuals, their families, and our communities are counting on you. Good luck!

The Jossey-Bass Health Series brings together the most current information and ideas in health care from the leaders in the field. Titles from the Jossey-Bass Health Series include these essential health care resources:

Curing Health Care: New Strategies for Quality Improvement, Donald M. Berwick, A. Blanton Godfrey, Jane Roessner.

Improving Clinical Practice: Total Quality Management and the Physician, David Blumenthal, Ann C. Scheck, Editors

The Juran Prescription: Clinical Quality Management, Kathleen Jennison Goonan, M.D.

Managed Care Contracting: A Practical Guide for Health Care Executives, William A. Garofalo, Eve. T. Horwitz, Thomas M. Reardon

Managing Patient Expectations: The Art of Finding and Keeping Loyal Patients, Susan Keane Baker

The New Health Partners: Renewing the Leadership of Physician Practice, Stephen E. Prather

New Rules: Regulation, Markets, and the Quality of American Health Care, Troyen A. Brennan, Donald M. Berwick

Physician Profiling: A Source Book for Health Care Administrators, Neill F. Piland, Kerstin B. Lynam, Editors

Profiting from Quality: Outcomes Strategies for Medical Practice, Steven F. Isenberg, Richard E. Gliklich

Restructuring Chronic Illness Management: Best Practices and Innovations in Team-Based Treatment, Jon B. Christianson, Ruth A. Taylor, David J. Knutson

Strategic Leadership in Medical Groups: Navigating Your Strategic Web, John D. Blair, Myron D. Fottler

The Authors

Samuel Forman, M.D., is chief medical officer of StatusOne Health Systems in Hopkinton, Massachusetts (www.statusone.com). He consults with a variety of organizations on improving the processes of care for their most seriously ill patients. Dr. Forman is active in the fields of population-based care management, disease management, and outcome measurement, topics on which he frequently lectures. Prior to embarking on his current venture, he led the medical management initiatives for the Health Centers Division of Blue Cross/Blue Shield of Massachusetts, where he demonstrated dramatic results with a forerunner of StatusOne. He previously led Procter and Gamble's health programs in North America.

Dr. Forman received his M.D. from Cornell Medical College and pursued postgraduate work in internal medicine at the National Naval Medical Center at Bethesda, Maryland. Additionally, he holds master's degrees in business from the Yale School of Management and in epidemiology from Harvard. He has contributed a number of articles to the peer-reviewed literature on clinical, epidemiological, and medical administrative topics. He is an adjunct associate professor of medicine at the University of Cincinnati Medical College.

Matthew Kelliher is president and chief executive officer of Status One Health Systems, Hopkinton, Massachusetts (www.statusone.com).

He is responsible for the overall direction, leadership, and marketing of Status One. He is directly involved with clients to ensure that their organizations realize the full potential of Status One services. Kelliher is an acknowledged innovator in the health care field. He successfully led organizations that initiated the first unconditional service guarantee, applied industrial quality control, and instituted manufacturing cost-accounting and redesign techniques that have provided industrywide breakthroughs in health care.

Prior to coming to Status One, as the executive director of the Health Centers Division of Blue Cross/Blue Shield of Massachusetts, Kelliher was responsible for the direction and profitability of this statewide capitated delivery system with over one hundred thousand managed care members. His experience also includes leading a pioneer quality management strategy as vice president at Harvard Community Health Plan, directing management-systems engineering at the University of California, San Diego, and consulting for Medicus Systems Corporation in Chicago.

Kelliher has a graduate degree in business from the Heller Graduate School at Roosevelt University and over twenty years of experience in improving health care systems at managed care organizations, academic medical centers, community general hospitals, and medical group practices throughout the United States.

Status One

Part I

....

Overview

1

High-Risk Population Health Management

No question about it, health care makes news. People care about it; they are even passionate about it. And, more often than not, the news about managed care portrays the industry as depriving patients in need of necessary care. Although this is not the whole picture, it is the perception many people hold.

At the same time, employers and government agencies that purchase health care services and the individuals who use them are not willing to pay for unlimited medical resources. Managed care organizations are constantly under pressure to lower costs by employers and government. Cost is not the only pressure however; purchasers and consumers of health care still want provider choice, broad access to care, and the latest technologies and therapies. The emergence of quality comparisons based on Health Employer Data Information Set (HEDIS) measures and National Committee for Quality Assurance (NCQA) accreditation is in response to these concerns. Federal and local governments are increasingly involved in mandating access, choice, and minimum lengths of stay (for example, legislatively mandated minimum lengths of hospitalization for childbirth).

The expectations for managed care organizations are exceptional. The current approach to meeting these expectations is not working. New ideas are clearly needed. One such approach, high-risk population health management, is based on stratifying the population to identify the very few people who are likely to require high-cost care in the near future. This population health management approach focuses on managing patients, not providers.

Achieving positive improvements in cost and clinical quality within this challenging environment entails rethinking how a managed care population is served. At the very least the health care system must address the peculiar needs of the highest-risk people, those whom we have labeled *Status One*. Rather than predominantly channel resources into credentialing, profiling providers, preauthorizations, and concurrent review (Kassirer, 1993b), this new strategy demands that care managers, providers, and the health care system proactively manage the medical care and related social and psychological support for the patients at highest risk. Rather than look for opportunities to deny care, with this strategy health care professionals search for ways to intervene quickly and to work collaboratively with the patient (Delbanco, 1992), family, and appropriate community resources to stabilize the clinical situation and prevent the need for high-cost care.

What Is High-Risk Population Health Management?

High-risk population health management is a new framework, or paradigm, for addressing the care of medically complex and chronically ill people. It is one of the few medical management strategies that can simultaneously deliver economic savings in the near term, benefit a problematic group, and serve as the foundation for improving care in the future for an entire population. This chapter provides an overview of key concepts and interventions, providing a basis for the more in-depth discussions that follow.

A paradigm is a way of conceiving the world. It is useful for understanding but may have the undesirable effect of limiting the scope of further learning, knowledge, and results. Kuhn (1996) cited a number of examples in his seminal work on the structure of scientific revolutions. High-risk population health management offers another way of viewing and serving a most challenging group of patients. Current managed care concepts do not adequately address the needs of this costly subset of the population.

Clinicians and administrators recognize that a small group of managed care patients require a disproportionate amount of resources. Although many believe that this need not be the case, no consensus has been reached as to which patients these are or which improvements and interventions will most benefit them. This is the challenge posed by the current paradigm, for it does not direct inquiry into disciplined patient identification, intervention, and program measurements.

What Distinguishes Status One Patients from Other At-Risk Patients?

Status One patients are at high statistical risk of deteriorating clinically and incurring high costs within the near term, usually the upcoming year. The members of this group can be predicted, they can be clinically managed, and their progress can be monitored.

The high-risk population health management approach entails identifying patients within a population according to the likelihood of both economic and clinical complexity and then adapting the provision of health services to the needs of each group. Status One patients, regardless of diagnoses, are most likely to incur high costs during the coming year and therefore command increased effort and attention. Ingenuity must be used to harness available clinical information and pharmacy and laboratory data to produce useful patient registries, while avoiding the impracticality that widespread use of chart reviews and questionnaires entails. Properly developed, clinical registries can be used like a laser to hone in on at-risk patient groups.

These high-risk, Status One patients often present the opportunity to understand patients' individual goals, involve them to the maximum extent their conditions allow, and improve the content and coordination of medical care. The right thing to do is to get things right for these, the most frail and needy, prior to embarking on yet another program for people in far better health.

Later, as clinical resources allow, the same kinds of methods can be used to extend care to additional groups at progressively lower risk for adverse economic outcomes. Stratification and early intervention with Status One patients constitute a unified strategy for systematically improving care across an entire managed care population. Stratification of a population and concomitant modulation of the intensity of interventions according to need is called population health management. Stratifying patient populations according to future economic and clinical risk is the cornerstone of population health management.

Even a cursory examination of the highest-risk patients reveals that they pose challenges most clinical systems are not ready to meet. For example, their complicated clinical situations defy care rendered during a typical fifteen-minute physician appointment, and the instability of their situation is poorly addressed by delays in getting appointments with specialists involved in their care. Yet the costs of not better addressing their needs are significant. Status One patients are complex both from clinical and psychosocial standpoints. There are relatively few, just 0.50 to 1.0 percent of the total population at any given time. Economically, each Status One patient costs ten to twenty times the average medical cost in a population (Forman, Kelliher, and Wood, 1997). Clinically, these individuals usually have more than one disease, called comorbidities, and acute episodes of care are increasing. No single, primary diagnosis accounts for more than 6 percent of them.

Status One patients are likely to become clinically complex and costly in the next year. The wide range of diseases found in the same people, who also are burdened with a variety of social-support and psychological challenges, results in a group whose chief commonality is that they are all different.

They are of all ages. Although seniors may be overrepresented in proportion to their numbers, those under sixty-five are usually in the majority. Their health problems typically isolate them from family, friends, coworkers, and community (Berkman, Walker, Boander, and Holmes, 1991). All too often a cycle of isolation, subclinical depression, and exacerbation of the clinical problems results. They tend to become increasingly dependent on the health care system and its highest acuity, most expensive components. This group turns over rapidly, 12 to 15 percent monthly, because of deaths, clinical improvement, or change in providers.

What Competencies and Resources Are Involved?

Competencies of population health management are the ability to *predict* who will benefit from care management, to *direct* efforts like a radar beacon toward efficient and preemptive care, to *customize* care planning to the needs of the patient, to *engage* the patient in restoring self-reliance, and to *monitor* outcomes on a population basis.

Resources include personal computers capable of linking to a secured intranet, registries of high-risk patients, a process for customized care planning, enthusiastic and trained case managers to help motivate individual patients, and a delivery system able to respond to the needs of high-risk patients.

Information on membership; provider; inpatient, outpatient, and emergency-room care; and drugs, which is found in all managed care organizations, must be integrated and analyzed on a regular basis to produce clinically meaningful patient registries. The Status One registry consists of the people at greatest risk of developing more severe medical problems and of increasing medical costs within the upcoming year. Case management tools deployed over an intranet link the patchwork quilt of modern health care systems and community resources into coherent care for individual patient plans. Intranets have a limited, defined set of authorized users, as contrasted with the publicly accessible internet. Case managers use these tools to support existing clinical care.

What Can Be Done Differently for Status One Patients?

No segmentation strategy or patient registry, regardless of how accurate and potentially useful, can achieve bottom-line results unless the process and content of care for high-risk patients are changed for the better. Health action plans are based on a patient-centered view that emphasizes the patients' goals and improves their autonomy and ownership. Plans are of short duration, in recognition of the urgency of the situation and patient instability. They foster the patient's involvement and autonomy, even in small increments. Something as minor as having the patient call the care manager with results of daily weight checks is more beneficial than having the same interaction initiated by a care manager. If the health professional initiates planned actions that the patient could have initiated as easily, an undesirable dependence on the health care system results. In addition, the delivery system needs to ensure timely access to care, communication and coordination among providers across the continuum of care, and forums in which health care professionals working with the high-risk population can share best practices.

In addition to improving the coordination of medical care, the traditional realm of case management, the assessment and health actions provide a systematic approach to dealing with psychosocial issues. Self-reliance, daily activity and fitness, interdependence with family and friends, mental challenge, and community involvement and purpose are all considerations in care plans for Status One patients.

What Distinguishes High-Risk Population Health Management from Traditional Medical Strategies?

Clinicians are trained to think of health care needs in terms of diseases and diagnoses. Each disease has a natural history. Some serious conditions, such as lung cancer, can be sharply reduced by removing environmental factors such as smoking and asbestos; whooping cough can be eradicated by childhood pertussis vaccination. Early, subclinical conditions can be screened for and treated before harm is done. Once the condition has been identified, it takes the form of a diagnosis whose natural history is known, and it is treated or cured. Established conditions can be treated in many cases. Clinical medicine can be conceived of as the quest for prevention, early intervention, and effective treatment. Health authorities label these strategies, respectively, as primary, secondary, and tertiary prevention (Last and Wallace, 1992). High-risk population health management is a form of tertiary prevention.

The single disease view is not helpful for tackling the dual challenge posed in managed care by the need to minimize cost and maximize quality across an entire population, particularly for the most vulnerable patients since most have comorbidities. High-risk population health management is a new concept on which to build population-oriented management strategies for medical care. It offers the framework for patient identification, intervention, and measurement of outcomes.

Current approaches to medical management generally have not met high-risk patients' needs. Case management was not designed to systematically predict who will benefit from additional services, and it does not track outcomes using the key metrics leaders use to manage the organization. Disease management works effectively for a number of patients diagnosed with a chronic illness, but it is often ineffective in the presence of comorbidities and psychosocial issues common to Status One patients. Organizations produce prodigious quantities of pathways and guidelines, call for large investments in clinical-data warehouses, and do not have the immediate impact or dedication required for the task. For many diseases, improved clinical outcomes may take years. Because no one disease accounts for more than a fraction of Status One patients, no one or few disease management programs can have a significant impact on this group as a whole.

Clinical quality improvement has borrowed heavily from industrial quality control theory, with an emphasis on conformance to "production" guidelines. This approach fails to accommodate the unique needs of Status One patients. High-risk population health management incorporates a variety of concepts from the quality movement—for example, developing health action plans to meet diverse Status One patients' needs based on the patients' priorities, a concept derived from mass customization (Oleson, 1998); and jobbing shop operations rather than using the production methods inherent in most disease management programs.

HMOs have not managed care but have succeeded in moderating cost by administrative efficiencies, contracting, and fee discounting. The low-hanging fruit are gone; the challenge, for which health plans are broadly not equipped, lies ahead. Cost rather than quality still drives the managed care marketplace. Organizations that want to stay competitive must improve the process of care for Status One patients. HMOs that do so have an opportunity to constructively engage with their providers by facilitating care for the clinicians' most problematic patients. As financial risk is increasingly shared or delegated to providers, such a collaborative strategy will be more and more welcome in the medical care delivery system.

Another distinguishing feature is that high-risk population health management aspires to refocus efforts toward managing care rather than providers. Providers and patients throughout the country are objecting to HMO medical policies that are inherently adversarial. Organized medicine speaks of the "hassle factor" (Bodenheimer, 1996) and garners legislative support to control it. It is not surprising. Managed care strategies that involved such administrative tactics as credentialing a network of providers, and arranging fees between the HMO insurer and the providers of care, have operated under the assumption that if you simply change incentives, not the system, meaningful operational change will follow. Today, too much of what is called "medical management" is based on systematic second-guessing and threats of vetoing payment for physician-recommended hospitalization, procedures, and drugs. Benefit structures derive from marketing studies, and coverage is designed for the majority of members or is determined by preferences of self-insured payers. This type of management was not formulated with the needs of Status One patients in mind.

What Will High-Risk Population Health Management Do for My Organization?

High-risk population health management will enable you, as a leader of a health care organization, to achieve cost savings through concentrated, proactive case management efforts that complement the usual clinical care. This paradigm offers health professionals the satisfaction of working creatively on behalf of an especially challenging group while achieving the near-term cost savings demanded by an unforgiving marketplace.

Who Benefits?

Patients benefit from improved access to care and attention to their condition, as well as from increased self-reliance in the face of debilitating conditions.

Reducing hospital admissions for the Status One group, thereby lessening their huge economic expenditures, can yield 2 to 5 percent bottom-line savings of overall medical costs. These savings can be applied to other clinical-improvement efforts benefiting a larger group of less ill people, to lowering premiums, and to increasing reserves or distributions to shareholders of the for-profit plans. In the fee for service (FFS) reimbursement environment, more complex care was always economically rewarding for all segments of the health industry. Under managed care, providers of the most *efficient* care are rewarded, at the expense of more costly alternatives leading to the same outcome.

Implementation Issues

High-risk population health management requires redesigning care for small subsets of challenging and costly members. The redesign effort is focused on creating more robust, proactive clinical processes that are responsive to the needs of the high-risk patient. As discussed later, health care leaders can anticipate and address resistance to altering the status quo. Redesign objectives include creating access, new services, and information-handling procedures that will meet Status One patients' needs. Table 1.1 relates the principal attributes of Status One patients to redesign objectives for the new systems of care.

Results

Measurement is important to gauge high-risk population health management. Population-based analyses require only a few essential measures that are meaningful to leaders and that reflect the care planning process and patient outcomes. Additional measures are of interest for research purposes but have little immediate value for program management.

• • • • • • •

High-risk population health management is the only medical management strategy capable of producing substantial cost savings and of having a positive impact on quality in the first year of full operation. Based on results published in the peer-review literature (Leveille and others, 1998), significant savings in an entire

Table 1.1. Program Design Implications of Status One Patient Characteristics.

Characteristic	Specification
At risk in the coming year	Efficient data availability for prognostication
	Predictive model
	Prepayment and risk-sharing financial arrangements
	Care manager and clinician education for new paradigm
Identified proactively	Systematic identification process using available data
	Patient registries
	Means of communicating information in registries to clinicians
Few in number	"Work-arounds" permissible rather than major insurance benefits and systems upheaval
	Clinician-identified patients can be added
Unique	Interventions robust across diagnoses
	Guidelines for particular diseases not pivotal
	Psychosocial issues incorporated
	Patient's motivators basis for action
	Health action plans customized
	Care planning resources and "curbside" consultations readily available
Deteriorating clinically	Care plans accessible across continuum of care
	Care managers have Status One patient panels
Unstable	Frequent registry updates
	Short-horizon care plans and reassessments
	Professional judgments on acuity and triage within Status One
	Care planning for as long as patients are at risk or until patient leaves system

organization's medical costs can be realized. It is fair to say that no organization has reached the limits of innovative care for Status One patients or of the performance impacts that can be realized. These are the kinds of results that can be expected in the chief programmatic outcomes (Forman, Kelliher, and Wood, 1997):

Reduce Status One per member per month costs by 10 to 20 percent

Improve functional status by 10 to 20 percent

Reduce Status One hospital use by 20 to 25 percent

Reduce overall medical cost by 2 to 5 percent

Part II

Components

2

· ·

Segmenting the Population

All managed care groups contain people in varying states of
health and therefore with health needs that differ greatly.
Linking people's perception of their health to how they seek medical care is necessary in both prepaid health plans and traditional
fee-for-service arrangements. With the managed care gatekeeper
approach, primary-care physicians use a variety of control procedures to limit unnecessary referrals to specialized, intense, and costly
services. In this era of increasing consumer knowledge, choice, and
activism, about 80 percent of all medical costs derive directly from
clinicians' decisions regarding necessary services (Eisenberg, 1986).
Clinicians often respond to their patients' requests, as the dramatic
introduction of sildenafil citrate (Viagra™) demonstrates. Physicians
can exhibit a wide range of variation in their clinical recommendations, a range unexplained by the best recommended therapies
from the medical literature (Wennberg, Freeman, and Culp, 1987;
Davidson, 1993).

Any cost and quality strategy must address either the need or
intensity of the most expensive services, which are typically hospital-based and under the direct influence of treating clinicians. For
the more severely or terminally ill, choices among complex therapy
alternatives remain difficult for a layperson to make. One medical
director holds his pen aloft in front of audiences and rightly declares

that it is the most expensive aspect of medical care. The pen is mightier than the sword when the holder also wields a stethoscope.

Concentrating efforts on the patients most in need is the most promising tactic in an era of renewed health care cost inflation, reluctant private and government payers, and shrinking insurer and provider margins.

Four-Quadrant Segmentation

Any big and complicated problem is easier to deal with in small parts. The same is true for the challenge posed by a managed care population. Breaking down a large membership into manageable pieces according to anticipated needs and to concentrate first on the most unstable and costly group is a cornerstone of the Status One strategy.

Segmenting a typical membership into four quadrants of perceived and objective health provides a useful division for conceiving medical management strategies (see Figure 2.1). It reveals a costly subgroup. Among them are Status One patients, whose needs are haphazardly met.

The four-quadrant model and quantitative estimates are based on our experience with capitated IDSs and health plans across the

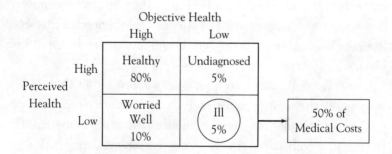

Figure 2.1. Segmentation of a Managed Care Population by Perceived and Objective Health Status.

©1998 StatusOne Health Systems, by permission.

country. The National Health Expenditure Survey has reported on the extent of perceived morbidity in the general population (Hoffman, Rice, and Sung, 1996). There is currently no published study in the peer review literature simultaneously quantifying managed care patients' perceived health, their providers' views of the same patients' health, and including subclinical conditions. The logistics of such a study done rigorously are daunting.

Simple condition prevalences would be insufficient for high-risk population health management. Essential hypertension may affect approximately 14 percent of a population, diabetes 5–8 percent, elevated cholesterol 10 percent, obesity 20 percent, cigarette smoking 18 percent, etc. What is important to our analysis and difficult to quantify precisely is to ascertain which of these conditions results in a patient having poor health *now* and how these same patients rate their own health *now*. For example, among the 5–8 percent of people with diabetes, the majority feel well and their providers consider their condition under control. Others may well have undiagnosed diabetes, unbeknownst to themselves or their doctor.

As a matter of developing a coherent medical management strategy, empirical evidence is sufficient and indicates the relative size of the four quadrant cells. The characteristics of Status One patients, as will be seen, are unequivocal. Both patients and providers agree that they experience impaired health. They are the least stable among this group, and—unlike the four quadrants—can be quantified and even predicted from existing data.

Questionnaires can ascertain members' subjective views of how they feel about their health. Among the most frequently used questionnaires are the Short Form 36 (Ware, Snow, Kosinski, and Gandek, 1995) and Probability of Repeated Hospitalizations (P_{ra}; Pacala, Boult, Reed, and Aliberti, 1997). Such tools typically contain a global impression of how the person feels, followed by assessments of daily activities, medication use, recent use of medical services, diet, and indications of depression. Chapter Nine gives further details on the varied ways to define high-risk groups. Regardless of the self-assessment instrument used, clinicians' views do not always coincide with members' reports regarding their own health.

The Healthy

Eighty percent of a typical population (plan, system, or community) is "healthy" at any given time as classified by both objective clinical criteria and self-reports. Whether the measures are inpatient admissions, ambulatory visits, prescription drug use, or self-reported functional status, the trend is clear. The majority of individuals feel, and objectively are, well.

Benefits such as health-club discounts and no-drug options in capitated senior plans are contemporary examples of plan designs targeting this group. HMOs have put a great deal of marketing effort into recruiting healthy members. A change in their numbers of a percentage point or two in either direction has a huge impact on overall medical costs.

Barriers to costly care, mid-level providers, clinical call centers, and precertifications are typical medical management tactics designed to get the right, modest amount of services for this group. Satisfying and retaining healthy people, who rarely require anything of the medical system, is both a necessity in order to spread actuarial risk with the ill and a challenge because of the need to provide inexpensive, valued services.

The Worried Well

People who feel ill, even though objective evaluations are normal, constitute a segment known as the "worried well" (Barsky, 1988). Physicians know them as frequent visitors to their offices and clinics. Some would earn the label of hypochondriac. Screening programs invariably attract them out of proportion to their numbers. They can account for a tenth of a typical population.

Limiting specialist referrals and requiring reasonable indications for elaborate diagnostic procedures are common tactics designed for the worried well. New, innovative programs to encourage alternative ways to wellness for this group show promising potential.

The Undiagnosed

Approximately 5 percent of a population does not think of themselves as having a disease or clinically threatening health issue, but in fact they harbor an undiagnosed condition. Depending on the aggressiveness of diagnostic screening, such diseases as adult-onset diabetes mellitus; essential hypertension; hyperlipidemias; cervical, breast, prostate, and colon neoplasms; and depression may remain undiagnosed for long periods.

Many HEDIS clinical measures evaluate diagnostic screening rates to detect such undiagnosed conditions, thereby singling out detection of common subclinical conditions. Despite the NCQA's representation of employers' interests in cost controls, the majority of spending is not on the undiagnosed, although this is a clear means of concentrating quality improvement initiatives.

The Ill and Status One Segments

The remaining 5 percent of the population account for 50 percent or more of all medical expenditures. A further subset, the Status

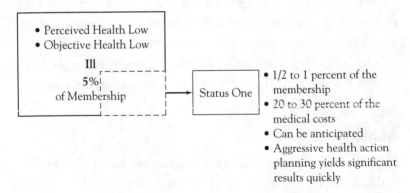

Figure 2.2. Ill and Status One Population Segments.

One group, consists of 0.5 to 1.0 percent of the total population but accounts for 20 to 30 percent of all medical costs. Their medical expenditures are, on average, ten to twenty times higher than average medical expenses. In a managed care population of 100,000, 0.76 percent of the population, identified prospectively, accumulated 24 percent of all inpatient admissions, 31 percent of all medical costs, and $2,284 PMPM (Forman, Kelliher, and Wood, 1997).

Attributes of Status One Patients

We have observed common attributes among Status One patients in a variety of managed care populations in different parts of the country. Statistical and epidemiological bases for identifying this group are discussed in Chapters Three and Fourteen. These are the pertinent aspects of this group as consistently found across delivery systems: they are at risk in the coming year for clinical complications and accompanying high cost; they are identified proactively; they are few in number; they have unique needs; their clinical situation is deteriorating; and their status is unstable. Some may be characterized as catastrophic cases, which insurers follow in large case management. Many more the providers do not even know about, a situation of particular interest.

It is useful to understand the characteristics of Status One patients. Doing so can provide a foundation for constructive interventions and allows us to appreciate how the needs of such a critical group can remain unmet by case management (Chapter Ten), disease management (Chapter Eleven), clinical quality improvement, and traditional managed care methods.

At Risk in the Coming Year

Because Status One patients are defined on the basis of future clinical complexity and associated high costs, opportunities exist to intervene constructively and to focus clinical efforts on those most in need.

High-intensity and high-acuity health care services drive high cost. Hospitalization is easily the most costly component of health care, though prescription drug costs are rising fastest on a percentage basis. Even in managed care delivery systems with the usual medical management strategies, Status One patients are being hospitalized at the rate of 12 to 18 percent each month. Fewer than a third have been hospitalized more than once in the preceding year, even though this is an often-used criterion for instituting case management.

Inpatient care is by far the highest cost component of all care. That is why managed care organizations rate each other by hospital admissions and inpatient days per thousand members per year. Typical plans have admission rates for the population under sixty-five of fifty to sixty per one thousand per year. In plans introducing a strong proactive orientation to Status One, high-risk patients will typically trend downward toward admission rates of forty to fifty per one thousand per year. Such results are useful Status One program measures as well.

Identified Proactively

Status One patients are identified in advance to allow time for meaningful clinical interventions to be effective. Available data include membership; provider; inpatient, emergency-room, and outpatient claims; laboratory results; dispensed prescriptions; and other information gathered expressly for the purpose of stratifying the population. Managed care and risk contracting have the advantage of having, at a minimum, administrative data from all health services delivered. An important advantage to using such data is that it provides a view of care in all settings and is identified in the same way from month to month, from one care manager to another. and from place to place.

Registries identifying Status One members to care managers and clinicians must be readily available. Registries provide a systematic, data-driven way to segment the population and to put the focus on those most in need of our attention.

Few

With fewer than 0.5 to 1.0 percent (that is, 5–10 per 1,000) of the population in Status One at any time, efforts can be sharply focused. In exclusively commercial populations, the prevalence of Status One members is 0.5 percent. Medicare elderly populations contain 1.5 to 2.0 percent Status One patients. In mixed commercial and senior managed care populations, of the kind served by general internists and family practitioners and including 10 to 15 percent Medicare risk members, the Status One prevalence is closer to 1.0 percent.

No single primary-care provider (PCP) has many Status One patients. No clinician should feel overwhelmed by the sheer number of Status One patients, but they are sometimes overwhelmed by the difficult task of managing these patients telephonically or through frequent but short office visits.

Unique

Social-support and psychological needs are common and rarely addressed. Isolation leading to subclinical depression is an under-lying contributor to high health care resource use in many situations. Assessments and health action planning get at these kinds of issues and are most effective when they involve the patients' priorities, aims, and desires (see Chapters Five, Six, and Seven).

It is common to have multiple diagnoses. No one condition predominates. Combinations of diabetes, hypertension, hyperlipidemia, asthma, emphysema, and other diseases often occur. The most common single diagnosis is congestive heart failure, but it is the chief diagnosis in only 4 to 6 percent of Status One patients. Given the multiplicity of psychosocial and clinical diagnoses, we can conclude that Status One patients are a small group of complex and challenging patients whose chief commonality is that they are all different.

Deteriorating Clinical Situations

Status One patients often have advanced disease states. Cure is frequently not expected. Learning to live with, and sometimes die from, a variety of conditions with dignity and the highest possible functional status is often the purpose of care planning.

The goal is to go beyond purely clinical care to break the cycle of isolation and depression that commonly leads to high-intensity care. Effective interventions engage the patient in the care planning process and change these unproductive dynamics.

Unstable

Approximately 12 to 15 percent of Status One patients are new each month. Similar numbers are discharged monthly. Patients newly appearing on a Status One registry will be maintained for as long as they meet the clinical algorithms predicting high cost and clinical instability. Patients are discharged when they improve enough to no longer be objectively and subjectively high risk.

People can be discharged earlier. Some die. Appropriate end-of-life planning is relevant for Status One patients who are terminally ill. Deaths range from 1 to 3 percent monthly. Some of the most gratifying interventions for patients and their families occur in the course of developing and implementing health action plans for terminally ill people, linking with and creatively engaging hospice resources.

Changing to a PCP outside the group or HMO plan and converting to indemnity insurance are examples of administrative reasons why people leave Status One early.

The efforts of the health care community must accommodate changing situations. Both short- and long-term positive results will be achieved through prompt, effective assessments and health action plans that are developed and customized with the needs of individual patients in mind.

Pathways to Clinical Excellence

The path to achieving clinical excellence within a population or community is becoming clear. Figure 2.3 depicts the qualitative road map to world-class results and robust processes through population health management. The axes track the period of time needed to improve clinical quality and expand a systematic and proactive approach to larger and larger segments of the population. Each of these phases is distinct and can be used to characterize the state of population health management within any managed care organization.

Random acts of clinical improvement, the first phase, is characteristic of most health care systems today. Typically, the health care system reacts in a fragmented manner—at times heroically, at times ineptly—to the needs of its members as situations arise. This phase is symptomatic of organizational paralysis; chronic problems are evident even to the patients, but a lack of organizational alignment and leadership prohibits real improvement beyond acts of advocacy and heroism practiced by front-line caregivers.

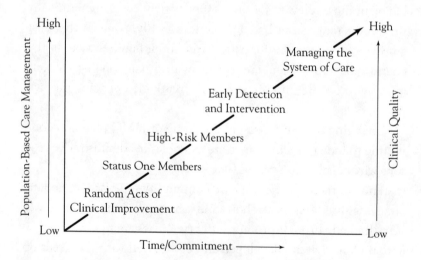

Figure 2.3. Clinical Pathways to Excellence.
©1998 StatusOne Health Systems, by permission.

Status One, the second phase, has a focused aim: to provide proactive, integrated care for the highest-risk members. At this stage, the aim for the managed care organization is modest in terms of the number of individuals affected but is vitally important. Specifically, to redesign the system of care for the vital few is an essential starting point for any population health management strategy.

Other *high-risk members* are the focus of the next phase of the population health management strategy. These members, although not as high-risk as Status One patients, are nevertheless an important aspect of a systematically expanding program. Segmentation of these members can be both by disease and by expected future cost. As always, separate registries will provide the platform for coordinating disease management and care management programs for these patients.

Early detection and intervention is the next broad phase of a population health management strategy. Using computerized screening criteria and historical clinical information, this registry identifies patients for proactive detection and intervention initiatives. However, rather than being ad hoc, this registry, much like Status One and high-risk designations, is routinely updated to include all patients needing designated interventions each month. Patients remain on the registry until the interventions are completed.

Managing the system of care is the pinnacle of population health management. In this final phase, all members within a population have a proactive health action plan. The plan is a contract for sharing responsibility among patient, family, and caregivers. Each member's action plan is focused on health goals for the next year. Although self-reliance is at the core of these health action plans, roles for the family, the community, the HMO, and the care-delivery system are integrated as appropriate.

• • • • • • •

Segmenting a managed care membership by perceived and objective health status reveals that the 5 percent who are ill account for 50 percent or more of all health care costs. Although 5 percent is a relatively small group, it is still too large to mount the most aggressive interventions. The ill group can be further segmented into the 0.5 to 1.0 percent of the entire membership who account for 20 to 30 percent of overall health care costs. They are a small but challenging group characterized by their future instability, uniqueness, clinical complexities, and psychosocial needs.

3

• •

Information

The Right Kind, in the Right Place, in Time

In this chapter, information strategies and tactics are discussed for identifying, managing, and monitoring subpopulations of high-risk patients. Our experience with the implementation of high-risk population health management is the source for many of the observations on obtaining the right kind of information, communicating it to the right people, and doing so in a timely fashion.

Population health management requires organizations to integrate data from various sources, transform the data into clinically useful information, promote knowledge-based collaboration for managing patient care, and ensure accountability for outcomes. For managed care organizations (MCOs) and integrated delivery systems (IDSs) that care for Status One patients, a good information technology strategy enables them to improve care for their most unstable members and provides a common platform for expansion to other at-risk populations. In addition, such a strategy links the patchwork of contemporary medical organizations together (Hagland, 1998), directly involves patients in their care, integrates community resources, and protects confidential health data (Computers, Science and Telecommunications Board, Commission on Physical Sciences, 1997). Information strategies can promote the use of clinical registries to define groups of patients for appropriate interventions and the use of the internet for disseminating information where and when it is needed. Any practical solution must be the least costly alternative for computer hardware, software, and communications investments.

Islands of Data

In order to begin to facilitate the care of Status One patients, information technology (IT) needs to bridge islands of data about individuals scattered among contractually linked health care providers and services. Care is fragmented, rendered by different clinical specialists and subspecialists in different places. This fragmentation poses a special challenge for Status One patients, who commonly see multiple specialists to treat their comorbidities.

At-risk patient registries may be based on questionnaires, existing data, electronic files, professional judgment, or combinations of these approaches. Accessing needed data is a significant IT challenge. Chapter Nine discusses various statistical methods for identifying Status One and other at-risk patients.

Case Example 3.1. Patient Data Needs

To put a human face on the discussion of technology, it is useful to visit a Status One patient and to consider him from the perspective of data-handling needs. Kenny Franco is a middle-aged male newly identified on the Status One registry. At five feet nine inches tall and 245 pounds, he is heavy-set and comes across as reserved. Diagnoses include non-insulin-dependent diabetes mellitus, obesity, and essential hypertension.

He was last hospitalized two years ago for diabetic ketoacidosis, which accompanied a viral gastrointestinal illness. He was on insulin while hospitalized. Presently he takes maximal dosages of oral hypoglycemic agents.

A workup for a diastolic blood pressure of 100 revealed compromised renal function with a serum creatinine of 2.1 and proteinuria.

Glucose control is poor as evidenced by 2+ glycosuria and an HbA_1c, a measure of long-term blood glucose control, elevated to almost twice normal at 11.2.

Several months ago an endocrinologist concurred with the PCP's longstanding recommendation to begin twice-daily insulin therapy. Mr. Franco refused, as he had since the hospitalization, saying that he did not want to deal with needles and injections. He has not seen his PCP in almost a year, anticipating a reprise of a stern lecture.

He was laid off from work because of his physical inability to perform his job as a machinist. Unable to obtain work in his trade, he is awaiting approval for Social Security Disability Income. He uses unemployment compensation and meager savings to maintain his HMO health insurance.

Mr. Franco had friends at work, but he is reluctant to contact them now. He used to like the outdoors and especially loved landscaping and gardening. He finds his excess weight embarrassing and has difficulty getting around. So he goes out rarely, only to the supermarket and movies. He is long divorced and has no children.

Mr. Franco, by seeking medical care in the most recent year from specialists, emergency rooms, and urgent care, is essentially lost to follow-up by his regular physician. Important facts about him are dispersed, effectively hidden among the interstices of the provider community, including hospital, emergency room, pharmacy, and clinical laboratory. No one in the provider community is fully aware of or takes responsibility for managing his deteriorating condition.

Relevant social information, including Mr. Franco's isolation and depressing living arrangement, his goals, and his reason for not beginning insulin therapy, have never been solicited, known, or recorded by anyone in the health care system.

These factors came to light only in the course of an explicitly targeted assessment process, described more fully in Chapter Five. The care manager worked out a health action plan with Mr. Franco that included planning and implementing a gardening project, thereby capitalizing on his love of working with his hands. A volunteer from a diabetic support group, who was also an active auto mechanic, stopped to visit and demystify the process of insulin treatment. A counselor familiar with Social Security benefits was able to help Mr. Franco understand his alternatives, which included state-supported vocational retraining programs that he was not aware of. By the time the care plan was reassessed eight weeks later, Mr. Franco had resumed regular visits to his PCP and was asking questions about insulin treatment.

This case demonstrates several aspects of how Status One patient care is critically dependent on gathering clinical and social data, integrating it, and linking the patient, clinician, and case manager to update the resulting care plan. A full explanation of the patient-centered assessment and care planning process is found in Chapters Five, Six, and Seven. At this point the focus is on IT.

Singling Out Important Patients

The challenge for IT is to use accessible data to single out needy patients for proactive care management prior to serious complications and deterioration of their health. For example, a typical managed care population includes thousands of diabetics. The American Diabetic Association asserts that 5–8 percent of Americans are diabetic. But during any given month only a small subset of diabetics are clinically unstable and at risk for catastrophe soon. The few people like Mr. Franco are thus of greatest concern to their providers and present the greatest near-term financial risk. Mr. Franco is a clinical disaster waiting to happen.

Precision need only go as far as identifying the likelihood of clinical instability and concomitant high costs. Important social and psychological information, useful for subsequent clinical interventions, usually is not documented anywhere and needs to be gathered separately, once a group of patients has been targeted. From a practical standpoint, such assessments can be conducted in-depth as long as they are focused on a small number of people most likely to benefit from proactive interventions.

Data Sources

Electronically accessible claims and pharmacy and laboratory databases are best suited for population health management and identifying Status One patients. Such data already exist and are readily available. The challenges are integrating data across payers and ensuring the timeliness of this information.

Electronically available data are not always as complete as data yielded by chart reviews, but chart reviews are resource-intensive. Figures 3.1, 3.2, and 3.3 illustrate the trade-offs involved. Figure 3.1 shows that higher-precision clinical data can be captured by investing more resources in retrieving and processing the information and presenting it to clinicians. The lowest cost and the easiest manipulations, however, are achieved by tapping into single, existing databases. By integrating such sources, data quality is improved but at an increased cost. Reviewing charts for the complex information needed for clinical use must be done by a nurse, whose expertise can be put to better use in the delivery of care. Compiling and presenting chart-review data require additional time and effort. Figure 3.2 indicates that as greater investments are made in gathering, integrating, and distributing automated medical databases, accessibility for clinical users improves. At the discontinuous point of switching to chart reviews, time for accessing data lengthens greatly. Status One monthly turnover rates of 12 to 15 percent therefore seriously limit the utility of chart reviews. The time delay between data gathering and registry production makes the information obsolete before it can be used. In addition, given the fragmentation of the health care delivery system, any single medical chart may not contain all the vital information required. Figure 3.3, which superimposes Figures 3.1 and 3.2, demonstrates that integrating existing automated

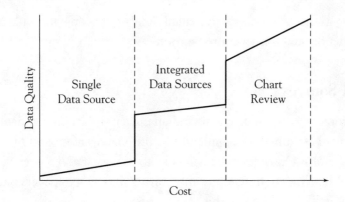

Figure 3.1. Relationship Between Data Quality and Cost.

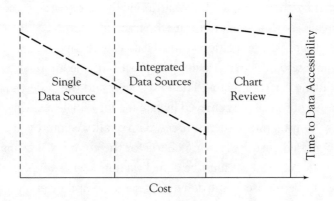

Figure 3.2. Relationship Between Data Accessibility and Cost.

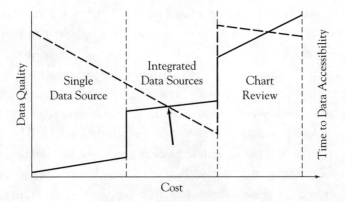

Figure 3.3. Trade-Offs Among Data Quality, Cost, and Accessibility.

databases is a desirable approach. Targeted chart review, done on a registry of high-risk patients derived from electronic sources, is fast, focused, and useful. It is the first step in the health action planning process for these Status One patients (Chapter Five).

Questionnaire data also require significant time and expense. Response rates are always a challenge with questionnaires sent to a broad audience. Coding, analysis, and dissemination add to the time from distribution of the survey instruments to return of the information to clinicians and nurse care managers. Again, the instability and turnover of Status One patients argue against reliance on questionnaires as a primary data source for identifying this group. There are also issues of how good a predictor of high costs questionnaires can be. Research (Coleman, 1998) has demonstrated the equivalent accuracy of electronic administrative data and functional status questionnaires filled out by the patient. Functional status questionnaires have the greatest utility in two situations: when they are used to obtain data on patients for whom there are no available electronic data, chiefly for new enrollees in health plans; and when they are the basis for care planning for a small set of patients already identified from computer-generated registries as being at risk. In these situations they are employed as diagnostic and care planning aids rather than as population screening tools.

Chapter Nine discusses the full range of alternative methods that can be employed to predict high-risk patients.

Predictive Models

Status One employs algorithms to produce registries of the highest-risk patients and specific, at-risk diseases. Algorithms for high-risk patients are predictive, meaning that they identify patterns of care that point to a deteriorating condition and significant future medical costs. Algorithms for specific at-risk diseases are descriptive, simply identifying these conditions in individual patients over time. The data run against these algorithms are from the previous twelve months. The output of this process is a registry of patients at risk for clinical complications and high costs during the subsequent year.

Most expert system algorithms of this type are proprietary. The reader may be disappointed but not surprised that such programs are not freely available in the scientific literature given the years of modeling and empirical testing involved in their formulation. Proprietary products are not new to the health care industry and are common in both clinical practice and management. For example, clinical laboratory kits, Disease Related Group analyses, inpatient severity-adjusters, and provider profiling software products all include proprietary components. Table 3.1 lists commercial vendors whose proprietary products include predictive modeling for managed-care populations. The list is necessarily incomplete because new firms are continually entering and leaving this field.

Leading and Lagging Indicators

Most algorithms are developed by testing countless combinations of leading and lagging indicators and deriving the optimal set capable of predicting high costs in the subsequent twelve months. Leading indicators are known prior to a disease exacerbation. Lagging indicators may have predictive value but appear after a clinical episode. The registry is updated monthly to accommodate patient turnover and the intrinsic instability of Status One patients.

In the case of Kenny Franco, the pharmacy prescription for the oral hypoglycemic metformin and elevated HbA_1c are leading indicators with respect to diabetic complications. A claim for emergency-room care is a lagging indicator in that it appears after a clinical complication has occurred.

Leading indicators include the following:

Authorizations for services

Pharmacy—specific drugs and route of administration

Laboratory values

Table 3.1. Commercially Available Models for Predicting High Cost
Patients from a Variety of Input Data.

Company	Contact Information	Typical Data Inputs
CareSoft, Inc.	1210 East Arques Ave. Sunnyvale, CA 94086 408-990-4700 www.caresoft.com	Health self- assessment
CareWise, Inc.	701 5th Ave., 26th Floor Seattle, WA 98104-7015 206-749-1100	Lifestyle risk assessments
Codman Research Group	138 River Rd. Andover, MA 01810 978-688-9318	Claims
CogniMed, LLC	70 Westview St. Lexington, MA 02173 781-674-2222 www.CogniMed.com	Claims
EcuCare International	100 Main St. Westbrook, ME 04092 207-856-6131	Claims
Franklin Health, Inc.	10 Mountainview Rd. Upper Saddle River, NJ 07458-1933 201-512-7057 www.franklinhealth.com	Claims
HBO & Company (HBOC)	301 Perimeter Center North Atlanta, GA 30346 770-393-6062 www.hboc.com	Claims
Health Decisions International, LLC	1667 Cole Blvd., 3rd Floor Golden, CO 80401 303-278-1700	Survey tool combined with claims
Healthtrac, Inc.	525 Middlefield Rd. Suite 250 Menlo Park, CA 94025 650-614-2638	Health-assessment questionnaire

(continued)

Table 3.1. *Continued*

Company	Contact Information	Typical Data Inputs
Heritage Information Systems, Inc.	410 West Franklin St. Richmond, VA 23220 804-644-8707	Claims
Johnson & Johnson Health Care Systems	425 Hoes Lane P.O. Box 6800 Piscataway, NJ 08854 732-562-3000	Questionnaire and measured biometrics
MEDai, Inc.	602 Courtland St. Suite 400 Orlando, FL 32804 407-644-5011 www.medai.com	Hospital charges, claims, and questionnaire
MEDecision, Inc.	724 West Lancaster Ave. Suite 200 Wayne, PA 19087 610-254-0202 www.MEDecision.com	Claims
ProMedex, Inc.	4301 Lake Boone Trail Suite 104 Raleigh, NC 27607 919-781-4533 www.promedex.net	Questionnaire
StatusOne Health Systems, Inc.	85 Main St. Hopkinton, MA 01748 508-497-9395 www.statusone.com	Pharmacy and laboratory claims, and questionnaire
ThinkMed, Inc.	312 East Wisconsin Ave. Suite 314 Milwaukee, WI 53202 414-287-6000 www.thinkmed.com	Claims

Radiology results

Genetic testing

Lagging indicators include the following:

Claims—inpatient and outpatient

Rehabilitation in a skilled nursing facility

Emergency room

Ambulance

Durable medical equipment

Renal dialysis

Questionnaire

These lists illustrate the range of clinically useful data that can be compiled from electronically accessible administrative and, when available, laboratory and pharmacy databases.

Individual paid claims include not only amounts but also diagnoses, procedures, places of service, and providers. By linking this information across time for every patient, we can begin to ascertain important clinical conditions and evaluate patterns of care. Although authorizations are made earlier in the treatment cycle than claims, they are less accurate than claims after they have been paid. Medical-record technicians expend considerable effort to properly use International Classification of Diseases (ICD) and Current Procedural Terminology (CPT) codes to standardize the coding for episodes of care. Inaccuracies creep in for a variety of reasons, but the fact remains that the data are already available and updated frequently.

Data "scrubbing" routines are required to cull out a variety of coding errors. Expectations for data precision are generally higher for clinical uses than for administrative purposes, even when considering the same data fields for the same patient. For example, an MCO and hospital may be content with a paid claim for a five-day hospital stay despite an ICD miscoding of the chief diagnosis as chronic obstructive lung disease instead of status asthmaticus. The implications for Status One identification and care are far greater. Using this type of data invariably results in falsely identifying a few people and likewise missing a few people who would be included if the source information were more accurate. Epidemiological sensitivity and specificity are discussed at length in Chapter Fourteen.

Some health plans and delivery systems have coded pharmacy and laboratory data available. Drug type and dosage can be a good marker for underlying diagnoses that would otherwise require laborious chart reviews. Insulin and oral hypoglycemics revealed by dispensed prescriptions are examples of efficient sources for construction of a diabetic registry, a job that would otherwise require an ad hoc scan of inpatient and outpatient visits and possibly laboratory data and a chart review. In contrast, matching pharmacy data to membership yields a fair picture of current diabetics under treatment, the type of information clinicians need to identify diabetics on their panels in order to plan proactive clinical efforts. Pharmacy data, coupled with outpatient and inpatient claims, are expected to challenge the accuracy of chart reviews and do so with greater speed and lower data-collection cost.

Clinical laboratory data are also useful in constructing and refining at-risk disease registries. Quantified test results are a useful source of leading indicators to complement claims information. For example, the fact that a claim for a hepatic antigen test panel was paid tells us only that a clinician was suspicious of the presence of hepatitis, whereas an elevated antigen titer is indicative of a specific type of hepatitis. When clinical registries are coupled with longitudinal patterns of care from claims data, accuracy can be greatly increased.

Most medical groups and plans have accessible pharmacy data for their members, and some have laboratory data. When both laboratory and pharmacy information are unavailable, predictive registries must rely on claims information to stratify the population; the registries then are less accurate but are still more useful than the unsystematic, traditional approaches.

Registries That Work

An essential component of a high-risk population health management strategy is the subpopulation-specific patient registries. Registries act like radar by scanning the population, locking onto and stratifying at-risk members. At-risk patient registries are the primary operational mechanism for stratifying patient panels into groups according to their likely needs. These registries provide a systematic means of transitioning from groupwide analyses to the care management of individual patients.

Status One extends the PCP or individual caregiver's field of vision. Registries assist clinicians and care managers in sorting population panels by likely need. Professional judgment, far from being minimized, is absolutely necessary to refine the registries and to encourage the patient to participate in clinical actions.

The physician and nurse care manager can define health action plans, just as an air-traffic controller files flight plans, but the patients determine arrival time and destination and pilot their own clinical course. Health action plans that are not contracted with the patient are unlikely to be executed or effective.

Caregivers need to be comfortable with the fact that at-risk patient registries invariably miss some people who do go on to having complex clinical situations and associated high costs. Also, some others who do not experience deteriorating conditions in the following year will be included. Despite these false positives and false negatives, at-risk patient registries extend the point of view beyond the horizon of immediate clinical experience. Most important, registries provide a standard system that can be monitored and improved over time. This more systemic approach to high-risk population health management is a great improvement over the current ad hoc, reactive approach to dealing with the patient at risk as crises occur.

Registries and Population Health Management

Registries provide a transition between epidemiology and clinical practice. Given a large population, they enable segmentation and focused clinical interventions. Properly executed, registries stratify a population for proactive care, for case and disease management initiatives. Without such capabilities, the clinician must wait passively until the patients arrive at the office. Likewise, case managers often rely on referrals from the physician. Status One patients, including those with the least stable and most complex conditions, frequently crash-land on the hospital's doorstep.

Registries have already earned their place in clinical practice. Oncologists and surgeons are familiar with hospital-based tumor registries. These registries maintain information on newly diagnosed neoplasms, tissue type, clinical stage, and course of treatment. Tumor registries have become a valuable source for determining the natural history of a variety of carcinomas and sarcomas, as well as the long-term effectiveness of new therapies.

Geographical disease registries have proven valuable in understanding disease patterns in a particular area and in comparing areas. The older such registries are, the more useful they are in improving the care management of chronic diseases. The Connecticut Cancer Registry and the Framingham Heart Study are two of the oldest and best known registries of this type.

Managed care recognizes additional benefits from the clinical use of registries. In order to increase prospective and preventive care, clinicians must understand the characteristics of the members of their panels. Unlike the historical use of registries for research and public health agendas, registries now have added significance and promise for improving the efficiency of patient care.

High-Risk and Disease Registries

Should patient registries be organized by disease or by intensity of resource use? The answer is both. High-risk patients cut across diagnoses, often have more than one condition at the same time, and have subclinical social and psychological problems. Other chronic-disease registries contain larger numbers of patients with greater clinical stability than Status One patients. The clinical challenge is to establish strong enough relationships with the Status One patients to allow coordination of clinical care and amelioration of the psychosocial factors that often lead to the highest intensity and costliest care. The Status One population should be effectively managed before the less severely ill at-risk patients in single-disease registries. Although most at-risk patients may be in more than one chronic disease registry at a time, if they rise to the risk level of Status One, our practice has been to list them only on the Status One registry until they stabilize clinically, change providers, or are deceased.

Useful disease registries that can be reliably derived from leading and lagging indicators are listed here.

- Endocrine

    Diabetes mellitus

- Neoplastic

    Neoplasms (excluding dermal squamous cell carcinoma)

    Specific neoplasms by type or site

- Musculoskeletal

    Degenerative joint disease

- Neurological

    Cerebrovascular accident

    Paraplegia

    Quadriplegia

    Spina bifida, meningomyelocele

- Pulmonary

    Asthma

    Chronic obstructive lung disease

    Cystic fibrosis

- Renal

    End-stage renal disease

    Chronic renal failure

- Gastrointestinal

    Cirrhosis of the liver

    Ulcerative colitis

    Regional enteritis

- Infectious and Immunological

    Hepatitis

    Tuberculosis

    Immunodeficiency

- Cardiovascular

    Atherosclerotic cardiovascular disease

    Myocardial infarction

    Cardiac arrhythmias

    Hyperlipidemias

- Psychiatric

    Depression

    Psychoses

Attributes of Patient Registries That Work

Registries must have a variety of attributes in order to be clinically useful. Epidemiologists may be tempted to immerse themselves in the intricacies of predicting outcomes in a general population from limited data. In truth, this is but one necessary step. In the extreme, a registry might be perfectly predictive but be so cumbersome and costly that it would be used rarely. For Status One patients such registries would be out of date within months and hence would lose their usefulness in helping clinicians focus their efforts on those who would most benefit from intervention. It is far more desirable to have a registry system that is reasonably accurate, inexpensive, and repeatedly updated with at-risk patients. Case managers must focus their efforts on optimizing the process of care and addressing unrecognized, subclinical social and psychological contributors to the patient's deteriorating condition.

Registries should thus be prospective in nature; easily understood as guides for determining medical management actions; frequently updated to reflect changes in health status and new information; inexpensive; timely; quantifiable in order to facilitate determination of their own accuracy; able to accommodate clinical judgment and overrides; capable of producing trended performance metrics essential to the success of the clinical enterprise; and consistent over time.

Delivery systems and HMOs charged with comparing competing approaches or with developing their own approach will find these attributes useful. (Chapter Fourteen discusses the various statistical methods available to construct registries: empirical triggers, multiple regression analyses, and neural networks.) At a practical level, care managers and PCPs will not care as much as leaders do about the machinery behind the registry "radar." Rather, they will be most interested in whether the registry works for them and serves as a tool to improve the care of their patients.

Prospective in Nature

The utility of a registry for identifying Status One patients depends on its prospective nature because Status One is defined in terms of future clinical complexity and associated costs. Status One patients are prospectively identified people whose conditions are most likely to become clinically complex and costly during a future interval. The future interval must be defined in terms of time and cost. The useful parameters for predicting Status One are a one-year interval and a cost of at least tenfold the average medical cost of the entire population. In fact, Status One patients can be categorized by any approach that prospectively identifies a small subset of the high-risk cases that will cost significantly more than the average.

Easily Understood

Any approach to high-risk population health management must be easy for the average physician, nurse, or social worker to grasp. Even if the most sophisticated analyses, clinical research, and computer technology are behind an approach, it must make sense to its front-line users. Using an auto analogy, no matter how fancy or plain the components under the hood are, what matters to the average driver is whether putting the key into the ignition reliably starts the engine.

Much of pharmaco-economics and outcomes research fails this test. Dollars spent per year of life saved, life-table analyses, and marginal benefits of one therapy over another in randomized clinical trials are examples of valid research outcomes not easily understood by clinicians and nurses pursuing their everyday practice.

High-risk population health management may be a novel concept, but it is straightforward for practitioners to grasp. Physicians can relate to the simple statement, "Doctor, these are your patients who seem to be at highest risk for hospitalization and clinical complications in the coming year." The challenge is clear and implicit: work creatively with the patient, family, community, caregivers, and the nurse care manager to get at underlying issues; devise a new health action plan; and avoid the need for complex and costly services.

Clinically Actionable

Registries fit into the clinical environment and as well provide a sound basis for monitoring population-based outcomes. A Status One registry, for example, invites immediate, proactive action. The care manager quickly initiates the assessment and care planning process.

The PCP can get right to work. "Do I know this patient?" "Have I seen her in recent months?" "Do I have a clinical care plan that is current and makes sense for the situation the care manager is evaluating?" Chapters Five, Six, and Seven detail the components of the care planning process.

Other at-risk disease registries provide the basis for direct actions supplementing ordinary clinical care without the need for ad hoc special investigations or chart reviews. And when such investigations are needed, they are far more focused and efficient than they would otherwise be. For example, if one wanted to be certain that chronic obstructive pulmonary disease (COPD) patients were offered the yearly influenza vaccine and had the benefit of pneumococcal vaccine prior to the winter season, the COPD registry would be the starting point for such a process. Employing the registries is an efficient approach to managing groups of at-risk patients.

Frequently Updated

Registries fit the clinical realities of those caring for at-risk patients only if they are current and up to date. Because Status One members are intrinsically unstable, no registry, no matter how accurately predictive, will yield any results that are of use to the provider of care unless it fairly reflects current risk profiles. Significant change in a patient's condition translates into changes in the risk profile and the registry. Future innovations in population health management will include instantaneous updates of relevant clinical data that will be distributed to authorized intranet users as soon as the data are known.

The less frequently registries are updated, the more outdated the information is and the more opportunities to proactively intervene are missed. Likewise, questions of data credibility will lead less to improving the care of individual high-risk patients and more to disputing the approach.

Kenny Franco will always be a diabetic and will be Status One so long as his near-term risk of complications is very high. Chronic-disease registries provide a means of quickly and constantly initiating disease management programs for patients like him. The need to link such registries to systems and programs for proactive care management is great.

Cost Effective

Practices or HMOs retaining financial risk must view the production of registries as a good value. Accurate but costly systems are not acceptable in the current unforgiving financial climate. Different organizations have different expectations for acceptable internal rates of return for clinical-improvement programs. Converting an organization's focus, direction, and competence toward population health management is not a program or project but a fundamental redesign of the basic business and vital to the organization's survival in the future. Most organizations expect financial benefits to accrue within a year of program initiation but may need to set their expectations on the longer term. The true test of the success of a population health-management strategy is that the health care system reaps the gains of preventing complex, costly illness.

Open to Clinical Judgment and Overrides

Clinicians rail at the notion of computers even suggesting how best to practice medicine. At-risk patient registries must facilitate and enable the clinical and care planning process. Surely each physician will have a few patients where intuition alone indicates heightened concern for adverse clinical events. The ability of registries to accommodate such patients is essential to clinician acceptance of a care management system.

Provider-designated patients enjoy the full benefits of proactive health action planning as part of the care manager's panel. However, such people should be separated in outcome measures to maintain the validity of comparisons across time and organizational units.

Another way to accommodate clinical judgment is to establish acuity levels, as described in later chapters. The care manager uses clinical judgment, together with the PCP's advice and personal knowledge of the patient and family, to anticipate when the need for hospitalization or some other intense clinical situation may occur. The result is an acuity level captured in the health action plan. It provides a means of melding professional judgments with system-generated registries. Benefits include continuous triage among the intrinsically unstable group of patients and a workload-balancing tool for leaders to use in rationally deploying resources where most needed.

Consistent Over Time

Algorithms for including patients in at-risk registries must be stable over time. Only new innovations in early detection or care management should be integrated into this forward control system. Although there is room for supplemental clinical judgments, when it comes to producing outcome metrics, only standardized inclusion criteria should be used. Likewise, this consistency forms the basis for evaluating proprietary algorithms and forward control systems likely to emerge in the technology market in the near future.

Care management methods that cannot define systematic inclusion criteria and report actual outcomes on this basis will fail to provide effectiveness measures over time. Additionally, the process will have no valid measures and, therefore, cannot be judged or improved objectively.

Enabling Knowledge-Based Collaboration

In the course of developing a health action plan for Kenny Franco, the care manager accessed several kinds of information. She initiated an informal, "curbside" consultation with a diabetes educator about the patient's refusal of insulin treatment, reviewed clinical guidelines on monitoring and providing therapy for diabetes and hypertension, and obtained information from the American Diabetes Association on community support groups. The PCP and endocrinologist each gave her input and advice about the care plan. The patient had access to this advice and other available knowledge bases in sorting among courses of action and choosing a few.

Information-handling strategies allow facts, advice, and opinion to be brought into the care planning process and to empower the patient. High-risk population health management encompasses these types of information:

- References

    Clinical guidelines accessible via an intranet

    Scientific literature available through hot links to authoritative sources like the National Library of Medicine and other clinical and health-oriented repositories

    Community resources

- Expert judgment and advice

    Case conferences

    Automated consultations

Ultimately, patients and their families can be fully empowered to plan their health care, make informed decisions, and commit themselves.

The Automated Medical Record

Since the late 1970s much creative work has been focused on automating the medical record (Steen, 1998). The vision has been of a paperless environment that enhances patient care by relieving providers of hard-copy recording chores and enabling cross-disciplinary collaboration. So far the results have not yet justified the investments. Some attempts have become bogged down because of tardy data transcription, cumbersome access of providers to terminals, legal requirements for paper copies and signatures, and the electronic inaccessibility of care rendered outside automated institutions.

Developments such as voice recognition, hand-held devices, power text search engines, and the internet will allow impressive strides to be made in the automation of medical records during the next millennium. Most important, the virtual medical record of the future must be fully shared with the patient online and on demand to support empowered, informed health care consumption.

• • • • • • •

Initially, an organization's high-risk population health management strategy for IT is to supplement, not replace, the medical record with ready access to the essential information from experts and references needed to care for Status One members, as captured and communicated on clinical registries.

4

. . . .

Structure

Building a Supportive Environment

This chapter is about building a supportive organizational environment to improve care for the highest-risk patients. This task entails readying case managers, primary care clinicians, systems specialists, and administrators to focus customized attention on Status One patients. Regardless of whether the organization is a group practice, independent practice association (IPA), staff-model clinic, or insurer, similar competencies will have to be built within the organization. Tactics may differ, but the essential challenge is the same.

Several group and individual roles important to changing the processes of care for Status One patients will be described, including steering committees and lead teams, care manager leaders, and clinical advisers. Case conferences and structured interactions involving the care managers are also described.

Prior chapters described how the population-segmentation strategy identifies a small and unstable subset of patients at the highest risk for clinical complications and associated high costs, while the IT strategy aims at handling essential information for their care across all settings. This chapter plows an organizational and personnel field in which improved care for Status One patients can flower into sustained improvements and efficiencies. Subsequent chapters delve into the care management process for individual high-risk patients.

Kenny Franco, the socially isolated, poorly controlled diabetic first encountered in Chapter Three, defies the rendering of good, integrated care. His needs can be neither thoroughly assessed nor fully addressed in the course of the typical fifteen-minute scheduled appointment, assuming he shows up for appointments at all. Clinicians who expand their time and commit the resources it takes to properly care for the Kenny Francos of managed care are few and far between. These exceptional physicians lack the supportive infrastructure needed and instead revert to random acts of clinical improvement to meet the needs of Status One patients.

Improving care for the highest-risk patients involves modifying the way care is accessed and delivered so that heroics and random acts are unnecessary. Fortunately, the very rarity of Status One patients implies that systems can be modified for them rather than redesigning care for everyone.

Several aspects of Status One patient care must be addressed structurally. Dedicated case managers supplement the usual primary and specialty health care. The infrastructure, people, and processes are aligned to direct the energies of these care managers, to place the full power of the organization behind their efforts, to integrate them into clinicians' practices, and to hold the entire organization accountable for meeting goals (Hanna, 1988).

A case manager is responsible for facilitating health action planning with the patient across the continuum of care and coordinating care regardless of the setting in which it occurs. Their aim is to decrease future health resource use and the need for future hospitalizations by increasing the functional status of individual patients. Comorbidities, clinical instability, and social issues require more thought, planning, and coordination than these patients ordinarily receive. Care management supplements and is closely coordinated with PCP activities.

Capitation and global risk encourage creative longitudinal care from an economic standpoint. Results come from addressing underlying social and psychological issues, enlisting patient involvement, and devising health action plans with the patient. Investments in predictive registries, case management, information systems, and outcome measurements are amply offset by reduction in the need for future hospitalizations and costly, high-acuity care.

Care Management Lead Team and Steering Committee

The care management lead team brings together people from the different disciplines that will be involved in improving the care of the highest-risk patients. It is empowered by the senior leadership to tackle this challenge as an integrated, systemwide project.

Some readers may share our bias against ad hoc administrative structures. Experience implementing high-risk patient management in disparate organizations has taught us that these or comparable permanent structures are necessary if the various clinical and administrative activities are to proceed in concert. Infrastructure, alignment, and key processes need to be in place before care managers begin formulating care plans with clinically and socially complex patients.

Some MCOs, IPAs in particular, have such diffuse clinical leadership that they should not attempt a project such as this unless they can develop leaders who can influence and drive the change throughout the provider network. Ironically, such organizations have been spearheading the assumption of financial risk, although some have no credible means for predicting and managing their highest-risk patients.

Team members include the medical director most responsible for the use of medical services, the leader of the care managers, a leading administrator, a representative from information systems, and staff selected to become care managers. Team members should be chosen not only for their existing authority in their MCO but also for their willingness to analyze and change the organization to serve the needs of Status One patients. Depending on how an organization is configured, additional members of the lead team could include leaders from home care, triage, scheduling, medical records, network development or provider relations, and clinical quality improvement if they are in a position to contribute to the team's goals.

An outside consultant can be invaluable in facilitating the lead team and supplying useful ideas from successful interventions elsewhere. We have an overt bias in favor of involving a consultant to assist with the breadth and depth of these tasks. The important thing is to recognize the essentials of what needs to be changed and to focus the organization on making these changes.

The lead team's basic responsibility is to work out a variety of clinical and administrative issues in advance, before the introduction of the high-risk care management program and before any care plans are devised. The lead team meets biweekly or more often in the initial phases to manage the many tasks and projects for which it has responsibility. As changes in care are effected, the team meets less frequently and can eventually be subsumed under established clinical leadership structures, usually within six months.

The care management lead team reports to a steering committee composed of the most senior clinical, administrative, and financial leaders of the organization. The roles of this committee include supplying adequate resources to implement the high-risk population health management strategy, removing barriers for the lead team, and holding the organization accountable for meeting its financial and functional status goals. Quarterly meetings of the steering committee are sufficient.

The steering committee and lead team should exist until effective health action plans are routinely being developed and carried out for the Status One patients and all key supporting processes have become routine. At that point the leadership of the organization should adopt population health management process and outcome measures as key data for monitoring the organization's practices and business.

Responsibilities of the Lead Team

The exact list of issues the lead team must deal with is derived from an analysis of existing processes and their deficiencies with respect to high-risk patients. A few issues and associated tasks that predictably occur in most places are described below.

Assessment Materials

Because assessing the patient's current situation is a key step in the care management process for high-risk patients (as further described in Chapter Five), documents to support care managers in conducting assessments of their patients must be created or adapted. These instruments include introductory letters to adult and pediatric patients who will participate in care planning, an age-appropriate health-assessment instrument that includes the patient's goals and social issues, and an initial health screen for telephone administration. Exhibits A and B are examples. (All exhibits can be found at the end of the book.)

The care management lead team reviews these forms, customizes them as necessary, and shepherds them through the appropriate organizational approval process. Often, a few physician advisers are able to review the forms and finalize them with the lead team.

The lead team has to determine how to produce, handle, and use registries for high-risk patients, and how to maintain and disseminate assessments and care plans; it also has to assist the care managers with the planning process via customized resource and consultant directories. We have supplied lead teams with a ready-made intranet application for handling registries, care plans, and communications. Any plan for high-risk patient care management will have to develop practical ways to supply assessment materials.

Experts

Consultants are identified experts in specific knowledge areas ranging from understanding disability benefits to managing diabetes to handling end-of-life issues. The reason for using them is to put the full weight of an organization's expertise into the care management process. These experts provide "curbside" consultations on key topics to care managers who provide a brief description of a patient situation and a specific question, usually via e-mail. Consultants are not expected to see individual patients, and the volume of requests for any one consultant is low. Most consultants are associated with a particular client organization, but if relevant expertise does not exist within an organization, a consultant from any location can participate. The care management lead team generally identifies consultants and then contacts the individuals to discuss their role, expectations, and how best to communicate with them. E-mail is preferred for groups capable of using it, because of its speed, directness, and informality.

Guidelines Selection and Links to Disease Management

The care management lead team is responsible for identifying clinical guidelines in use in the organization and making them available for high-risk care planning. Guidelines, as Chapter Six explains, are common in clinical-improvement programs. Most delivery systems and insurers have several, most often ones they have invented themselves, adopted from external organizations, or combined from internal and external sources.

Status One patients, because of their comorbidities and social complications, are exceptions to clinical guidelines. Portions of a guideline may be useful as a reference for some aspect of their care, but not the guideline in its entirety. The recommended tactic is to capture an organization's favored clinical guidelines into the care management process but to avoid launching groups to create new ones expressly for Status One patients.

Customized Directories of Ancillary and Community Services

One of the key implementation activities of the lead team is to compile resource directories of the community and health services available in the local geographical area. The resource directory lists community organizations able to fulfill a myriad of needs of high-risk patients; they can supply transportation, home care, durable medical equipment, meals, and references to support groups and chronic-disease associations.

A separate education and fitness directory lists a variety of activities including arts, music, fitness, and special-interest classes; walking groups; exercise classes; fitness centers; and personal trainers. These groups are based in the community and accessible to high-risk patients. These two directories are extremely helpful to care managers in providing options to patients when developing their individualized care plans.

Data Handling

The IT representative on the lead team is responsible for identifying electronically accessible claims and, if available, pharmacy and laboratory data from which the predictive registries will be derived. Organizations creating their own predictive algorithms and data flows that will culminate in routine production registries will need time and resources to create this data warehousing and analysis function. Without it, highly focused care planning cannot proceed systematically. Chapter Three described outsourcing opportunities for population-based data analysis.

In addition, the lead team ensures that care managers have the hardware they need, including computers, modems, and intranet access, for using care management software and accessing the community ancillary resource lists and consultants. Developing a system for issuing passwords for automated systems as well as ensuring hard-copy security are important tasks for the lead team.

Training

Another of the tasks overseen by the lead team is the training of care managers, PCPs, consultants, and selected specialists.

The most intense and time-consuming training is for care managers. Care managers are central to the success of high-risk population management. They "quarterback" the new process for this small group of patients. They are trained to understand the concepts behind population-based risk stratification, to explain the importance of managing Status One patients to the organization, to use a common care planning approach that merges clinical and psychosocial models, to become proficient in using supporting technology, and to devise and implement health action plans. This training certifies the care managers' skills prior to their contacting patients.

A great and undesirable variation in preparation prevails in the professional nursing and social work communities. Such variability can be seen even within a single institution. Care managers also tend to work without a systematic way of sharing key resources and experience with colleagues. A brief training program covering the aforementioned issues establishes a common understanding and increased capability among care managers.

A great deal of the success in working with Status One patients depends on what happens at the point of care. Therefore, it is critically important that staff directly involved in meeting patients' needs participate in an orientation to Status One care management. The orientation should cover the importance to the organization of managing this small population closely, the concepts of high-risk patient management, the value of integrating the psychosocial needs of patients with their health care, and the care planning process. PCPs, each of whom typically has a handful of Status One patients, learn about the resources the care managers bring to high-risk patient care, respond openly to requests to optimize potential gaps in medical care, and designate their own high-risk patients for care management. Such referrals increase provider acceptance and serve an important function in augmenting computer-derived Status One registries.

Not only is the Status One message clear, it is also appealing. The transparent aim, to supplement traditional care with an aggressive and anticipatory brand of care management, is the opposite of those aspects of managed care so abhorrent to care providers: prior approval, second opinions, concurrent review, benefit caps, and other barriers to care.

After orientation, PCPs need to have direct interactions with care managers and involvement in case conferences to reinforce new practices. Clinicians learn best in discussions about improving care for some of their most challenging patients.

Generally, the same materials used to orient the physicians and staff will help the consultants prepare for their role in supporting the care managers working with Status One patients. In addition, the role description for consultants and what is expected of them should be clarified in an orientation session for them.

Clinical Case Conferences

The lead team may have to introduce or redirect clinician meetings in order to obtain a sustained focus on the highest-risk patients. Case conferences are discussions about particular Status One patients among colleague PCPs, the care managers they work with regularly, and allied services such as home care and pharmacy. The focus of the case conference, depending on the case, can be to share a best practice for high-risk patient care, solicit ideas for a particularly challenging situation, or alert colleagues about a complex patient they may be covering.

Practices will discuss different kinds of situations in case conferences. Some IPAs and groups have utilization rounds, where opportunities to avoid long hospitalization stays and to review referrals are discussed. These rounds can be adapted to the more proactive Status One process. In organizations in which physicians are "practicing alone together," physicians seldom convene to discuss the practice of medicine. Instituting case conferences in these settings requires strong clinical leadership.

An insurer works at a disadvantage relative to an IDS for purposes of Status One case conferences. The risk-bearing IDS is a more fertile field for case conferencing than an HMO insurer. The HMO insurer is most often one payer to nonexclusive providers.

Rarely will enough Status One patients be concentrated in one office practice to justify frequent conferences unless conferencing is combined among a number of PCPs and facilitated by the regional medical director.

When adopted as a lead team strategy, case conferences should be held weekly or biweekly and should comprise physicians actively practicing together—for example, a community practice in an IPA or a pod of internists and family practitioners within a larger group-model setting. If conferences occur as infrequently as every month or if large clinician groups meet together, they assume a grand-rounds type of didactic atmosphere, a situation that loses the immediacy and clinical importance found in small groups of clinicians who have a high likelihood of actually caring for the patient being discussed.

Clinical Advisers

The care management lead team should appoint a clinical adviser to coach and encourage the care managers. In a risk-bearing insurer, an associate medical director who is actively seeing patients would best fill this role. In delivery systems the clinical adviser could be a clinically active medical director or an influential PCP from among component practices. Insurers may identify part-time associate medical directors, selected from among practices with large numbers of that insurers' patients, to serve as clinical advisers to their care managers. For clinical advisers to be accepted champions, they need to be in active practice for the majority of their time, part of the delivery system, and respected by it. Additionally, the clinical adviser should be an active advocate for the conjoined clinical and psychosocial model of care for the highest-risk patients and should become proficient in the mechanics of health action planning and the use of technological supports. Training of the clinical adviser can be supplied in the training seminar for case managers.

The clinical adviser fosters a learning environment by providing physicians with a sounding board for complex situations; this relationship supplements the chief interaction between the care manager and the patient's PCP. In addition, the adviser calibrates judgment calls in the care of Status One patients and intervenes as clinical ombudsman in regard to occasional provider misunderstandings and lapses. One clinical adviser can comfortably interact with three to five care managers during one clinical session per month.

Individual Care Manager Interactions with PCPs

Care managers must be afforded the opportunity to interact with PCPs and heavily utilized specialists. The steering committee may need to influence organizational policy and administrative practice to enable professional collaboration.

As will be seen in Chapters Five and Six, issues regularly arise concerning introducing the care manager to new Status One patients, refining aspects of medical care, and jointly devising input to the care plan. In these discussions the PCPs can add high-risk patients they feel the predictive algorithms have missed.

Collaboration between care manager and clinician may occur during scheduled meetings, phone conversations, or unscheduled hallway meetings. Unscheduled meetings may suffice in small clinics where the care manager is physically located, while scheduled meetings require deliberate planning. Insurers should consider reimbursing providers for the time spent in such planning on behalf of their HMO-insured Status One patients if the providers do not share risk. However these interactions take place, they are far too important to the patients and to MCO finances to be haphazard.

Benefit Exceptions

The care management lead team must define a fair and viable policy for making benefit exceptions when they are important to Status One patient care. Most often exceptions are not the expensive, extracontractual items for which insurers already have procedures, but rather they are minor items such as babysitting or taxicab fare, the absence of which contributes to high-risk situations by making it difficult for patients to see providers and obtain needed care. A Status One approach requires resolutions to these difficulties to be worked out in advance, to be liberally applied, and to be easy for the care manager to invoke.

Unfortunately, most insurers have designed their benefit plans for the average subscriber. Status One patients clearly do not fit this mold. Insurers tend to become bureaucratic and legalistic to avoid making exceptions, fearing a torrent of subscribers demanding that the benefit extended exceptionally to a Status One patient be given to all. Others fear that the NCQA will take offense at irregular benefit administration.

This stance calls to mind the misguided hunter who shoots at the mice while the elephants run by. Experience shows both concerns to be misplaced, calling attention to small issues while needs go unmet and medical costs become elephantine. Exceptions are already made through an orderly process. Being the highest of the high-risk patients is reason enough to extend an unreimbursed benefit if it is part of a care plan aimed at maintaining the patient's functional status and reducing the need for costly, usually inpatient, care. To deny what is needed now results in far higher costs soon enough.

Delivery systems at financial risk have a much easier time with exceptions. Often creative enlistment of community and disease interest groups for free precludes the need to spend more. When a situation is not covered by the insurer's benefit package, the delivery system has every incentive to do what it thinks is correct for the patient. A risk-bearing delivery system will find ways to get around restrictive insurer interpretations. One system we know of insists in the insurer's presence that they make no benefit exceptions but do concede they do "favors" for the rare patient in need when the delivery system is fully subcapitated for them.

Reaching a Steady State

When the first Status One registry appears in an organization, each care manager may suddenly find herself or himself with a panel of fifty high-risk patients to manage. In a steady state, a care manager will have to start up only about five to eight new patients in a given month, so getting fifty going all at once is overwhelming. The lead team and the line organization of the care managers need to design a start-up plan that brings care managers up to their full panel size systematically and as quickly as possible.

A start-up approach designed by the lead team and line organization is selected and communicated to the care managers, physicians, and other designated staff. Once the initial registry is produced, the care managers embark on their work by ramping up according to the selected approach.

Several start-up methods have been used successfully. Building the registry block by block has worked for organizations having multiple managed care payers and receiving the necessary data at different times. If the claims and eligibility data happen to stagger in, a smaller registry is generated initially. The registry grows over a few months as incremental payer data is added.

Others have allocated and trained temporary help. An organization's own triage nurses or an outside agency places the initial health-screen calls over a short period of time. These calls enable the nurses to set an acuity level for triaging among Status One patients. The care managers then work on the most clearly at-risk patients followed by the next priority level and so forth until care plans have been developed for the entire Status One registry.

Another approach is for care managers and the PCPs to prioritize each panel. Following an orientation for PCPs, each care manager meets individually with each of the PCPs to review the physician's registry of Status One patients. Together they prioritize the registry to attend first to the patients the physicians know have an urgent need, then to assess the patients unknown to the PCP, and lastly to begin working with the patients the physician knows but about whom the PCP is less concerned. The risk in the approach is that the acuity assessment is made without current information on clinical condition from the patient.

. . . .

In this chapter a structure conducive to the care of the frail and unstable was described. Ultimately responsible to a leadership steering committee, the lead team tackles a variety of tasks including training, data collection, resource and guideline identification, and benefits exceptions. The new role of clinical adviser is adapted to provide a medical sounding board for the care managers. Organizational policies facilitate the collaboration between provider and care manager. The aim is to place the full force of a clinical organization behind proactive care of the small but challenging Status One population.

5

Assessing the Patient

Getting to the Heart of the Matter

Care management for Status One patients should be a core process for MCOs to master in order to meet the needs of high-risk patients in the present and to position themselves for further population-based approaches. No matter how accurate the stratification process is in identifying Status One clients, any initiative that focuses on assessments and identification of at-risk patients while neglecting practical improvements in their care cannot yield results.

This chapter focuses on best practices for assessing high-risk patients as a prelude to customized interventions. Previous chapters have discussed Status One strategies in population-based care management, stratification of the managed care membership, strategies for IT, and structural changes for achieving breakthrough results. Deficiencies in current case management are the subject of Chapter Ten. A full understanding of case management as it is currently practiced is indispensable when leading change in an organization. Deficiencies in current methods cannot be carried into population-based health management if one intends to have a positive impact on at-risk patients over time.

Patient Identification

The start of the care planning process is the appearance of a client on the Status One registry, which is updated monthly. The registry of Status One patients predicts those most likely to need high-cost, high-intensity medical services in the near term; it forms the basis for proactive care management. Although complex in some respects, the identification process should be invisible to the care manager, much as an ambulance driver does not second-guess presenting symptoms when an emergency call is made. Rather care managers perform an assessment of all Status One patients to establish an appropriate treatment and plan.

There is also a place for professional judgment. If the PCP or care manager judges that additional patients will become clinically unstable and costly during the near term, they are added to the Status One registry. This process applies also to newly enrolled members in whom the enrollment questionnaire or introductory visit indicates clinical instability. Absent experience with which the predictive computer algorithms could identify them, these clinically unstable new members also are added to the highest-risk group and benefit from the full range of proactive care management services. Physicians will add approximately 5–15 percent to the registry size, a feature of value both to the patients benefiting from added attention and to clinicians, who gain an extra hand in the care of their most challenging patients.

As a matter of nomenclature, the Status One member is identified both as a patient and as a client. This distinction is often cited in the nursing literature. It is important to some nurses and social workers to differentiate their clinical interactions from those of physicians. Status One members are *patients*, in that clinical conditions require them to be actively under a physician's care. They are simultaneously *clients* and will be part of a panel followed by the care manager for as long as they appear on the Status One registry.

Assignment of a Care Manager

Each Status One patient should have a single care manager for the duration of his or her sojourn on the highest-risk registry. Each care manager carries a panel of forty to sixty Status One clients and assumes primary responsibility for care planning across the continuum of settings. Each PCP is assigned one care manager in order to facilitate collaboration. Care managers support several PCPs, whose Status One patients in aggregate fill the care manager's panel.

The process depends on prompt assignment of new Status One patients to their care managers. The patients are intrinsically unstable. Prior to effective care planning, 15 to 18 percent of Status One patients will be hospitalized each month. Needless delay in assigning care managers or at any other stage in the assessment and intervention phases invites further complications to occur and provides no chance of avoiding them. A phrase that summarizes this necessity emerged from an early implementation: "If the wages of sin are death, the consequences of delaying care for Status One patients are hospitalizations and complications that might not have occurred." The wording and dire consequences seem biblical, but it does capture the sense of urgency to speedily assess and engage new Status One patients.

Patient Assessment

Direct client contact is the gold standard for Status One care planning. It would be difficult to conceive of fully engaging a person in the psychosocial Status One aims if that person is only a disembodied voice over the phone.

The purpose of assessment activities is to clarify the current situation from both client and clinical perspectives, and to develop a trusting relationship among care manager, patient, family, and the delivery system. Assessment identifies which of the Status One aims, as detailed in Chapter Six, will likely become part of the health action plan.

Keeping several principles in mind sets the stage for maximum engagement and collaboration with the client. These include: (1) clients are active participants in the process and are capable of managing their health; (2) the object of assessment is to capture the *clients'* priorities and to ascertain which health actions they are likely to commit to. Motivational interviewing is uniquely suited to meeting these goals (Miller and Rolnick, 1991).

The recommended assessment sequence begins with a quick review of the case background from the medical record. This review familiarizes the care manager enough with the case to grasp the client's major diagnoses; the care manager can also note the most recent time the client has had contact with the PCP.

Next, a letter of introduction from the PCP (Exhibit A) is mailed to the client with a health assessment questionnaire. The letter introduces the care manager as an agent of the PCP, and the health assessment questionnaire obtains functional status information that will become useful for incorporating the client's perspectives into care planning; this information is not otherwise available in the health records. The PCP's signature on the introductory letter enables the care manager to act on behalf of, and as an extension of, the patient's physician. If it is impractical to obtain the PCP's signature, the care manager should obtain their permission to proceed with the assessment and mention this in the letter from the care manager to the patient. The conversation between care manager and PCP at the outset of Status One patient assessment sets the stage for all subsequent activities. From the beginning, the clinician is involved in Status One care management. Additionally, potential concerns of the patient, clinician, case manager, or observers are allayed.

Case managers employed by the insurer and not actively working with the clinician must engage the PCP in order to pursue the most aggressive care management strategies. An important aspect of readying the risk-retaining HMO for population-based health management of its highest-risk Status One members is aligning care-manager activities closely with the network of PCPs.

Existing assessment questionnaires have minimal psychosocial information and hence must be extended to cover the Status One aims. The health assessment questionnaire includes general thoughts on health status, social involvement, mobility and fall risk, nutrition, substance abuse and smoking, depression, and planning for the future (health-care proxy, living will, advanced directives). These parameters are included in many functional status questionnaires (for example, Ware, Snow, Kosinski, and Gandek, 1995) with the exception of several of the psychosocial domains and patient's aims.

It is important to distinguish use of health assessment questionnaires from population-based screening. The questionnaires are used as the basis for care planning for individual Status One clients. It is a clinical use rather than membership screening, as in the validation research for the Ware's SF-36 and SF-12 surveys. The Status One health assessment questionnaires are used to gain information on lifestyle and priorities from people already at high risk according to the predictive algorithms. They are not employed to stratify a broad population but rather to work up individual care plans.

Right after the introductory mailing, the care manager calls the client to introduce herself or himself, to reinforce the usefulness of the health assessment questionnaire, and to set up a meeting (Exhibit B). In order to encourage self-reliance, the client should come in to see the care manager. Often this visit can be arranged on the same day as a scheduled physician visit. The call also allows an initial estimation of the client's acuity, a triage estimate by the care manager of the client's relative stability.

When making the initial call, the care manager must be prepared for the exceptional situation (see Table 5.1). Language issues, mental incompetence, mobility limitations should all be known and accommodated early in the assessment process. A visit to the home should be made by the care manager or home-care agency acting in the care manager's behalf only if an office visit is not feasible. If the

Table 5.1. Approaches to Exceptional Situations During the Initial Call and Health Screen.

Situation	Approach
Incompetent	Talk to companion or chief care giver
Language barrier	Obtain translator—close family member best
Can't get through	Request in-home assessment
Refusal	Keep trying. Proceed with comprehensive medical care review
Deceased	Express empathy

patient has passed away between appearance on the registry and the initial call, expressing condolences to the grieving family is appropriate. Family members can see such a contact as a humane expression from the clinical care team, although it is frustrating to the care manager, who had expected to help a living person.

Assessing acuity levels enables care managers to triage the Status One registry, an important consideration for an intrinsically unstable group. Acuity is updated by the care manager and should be modified on the basis of the most current information. Acuity levels are defined as follows:

Level 1: Expect hospitalization in the next one to three months

Level 2: Expect hospitalization in the next three to six months

Level 3: Expect hospitalization in the next six to twelve months

Level 4: Expect hospitalization in the next twelve to twenty-four months

Level 5: Expect hospitalization in the next twenty-four to thirty-six months

Additionally, an assessment of functional status, the client's global view of his or her well-being, is also a useful triage strategy.

The question usually asked is, "Considering everything, how would you rate your health?" or "In general, how would you say your health is?" The client is asked to respond on a scale of 1 (poor) to 5 (excellent). A client's report of poor health is a red flag in itself of potential clinical instability.

The brief functional status assessment also serves as the basis for a useful population-based measure; the population aggregate can be interpreted over time in comparison with baseline levels as a measure of the effectiveness of care planning. Similar questions appear in the initial health screen by phone and the health assessment questionnaire.

An in-home assessment is an optional means of clarifying important issues, dealing with a shut-in, furthering personal rapport, or completing the health assessment questionnaire if it is not obtained by mail. The care manager, the Visiting Nurse Association, or a senior-community-services representative could make the home visit, depending on availability and close alignment with the Status One care management process. We recommend in-home assessment as a second-line tool in order to avoid the client passivity that a "we'll-come-to-you" approach engenders.

Comprehensive Medical Care Review

The comprehensive medical care review is part of assessing a newly identified Status One patient. The review is based on the medical records and clinicians' assessments. These are the sources for performing a comprehensive medical care review:

Medical record

Problem list

Medication list

Outpatient visits

Recent inpatient discharge summary

Psychiatric record

Home-care notes, if on service

Records of rehabilitation in a skilled nursing facility or long-term care records

PCP, specialist discussions

Although case managers often view optimizing the coordination of medical care as their domain, interventions on behalf of Status One patients demand a new perspective. Traditional case management often seeks to understand and carry out physician orders as part of hospital discharge planning. Status One assessments require review of clinical care in order to identify a variety of potential gaps and omissions. If important aspects of medical care have already been identified, they will be prioritized, negotiated with the patient, and become part of the health action plan.

It is more difficult to assess the clinical situation for errors of omission than for errors of commission. Reference to clinical guidelines, discussion with the PCP and involved specialists, and informal consultations are often necessary to fully assess clinical care in a complex situation. In Chapter Three, programming for intranet-based care management software was described. Encompassing clinical guidelines, hot links to authoritative internet web sites and local experts who have agreed to support Status One health action planning via electronic mail, this software facilitates assessment and planning by making expert knowledge and judgments readily available. Such activity supplements the primary- and specialty-care knowledge applied to Status One patients and accessible in the medical records.

Figure 5.1 outlines the seven areas in which important gaps in medical care may occur: physician involvement, access,

Patient involvement

- Information not shared by providers and patients
- Patient inquiries not answered
- Missed opportunity for education
- No pharmacy involvement
- No sharing of triage and urgent-care points of contact with patient

Process of care

- Patient seen primarily in emergency room or urgent care, or as inpatient
- Patient back for repeat visits without resolution or plan
- Repetitive tests
- Unaddressed opportunities for home care
- Disease guidelines not used

Care providers

- Lack of PCP involvement
- Lack of appropriate specialty involvement

Coordination of care

- No clinical care plan
- Care not integrated among providers
- Uncoordinated treatment
  - Anticoagulation
  - Insulin
- Advanced directives not in place

Documentation of care

- No updated problem list
- No updated medication list
- No current plan of care
- No discharge summary from recent hospitalization

Access to care

- No regular schedule
- Waiting too long for access to:
  - Primary-care provider
  - Specialty-care provider
  - Diagnostic testing
- Transportation, child-care barriers
- Telephone help not available twenty-four hours a day

Follow-up

- No follow-up on key abnormal laboratory tests
- No regular provider follow-up to episodic emergency-room or urgent care
- No follow-up on care plans

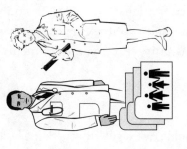

Figure 5.1. Gaps in Care as Identified in Comprehensive Medical Care Reviews.

coordination, process, documentation, patient involvement, and follow-up to episodes of clinical care.

Care Providers

PCP involvement may be absent. PCPs are often unfamiliar with many of the patients on the Status One registry. The reasons are as disparate as missed appointments, exclusive use of emergency rooms (ERs) for care, and new membership.

Specialists may be driving the care, an appropriate situation for people with active neoplasms and for end-stage renal disease. In situations where specialists are dominating the care, it is important that they assume the PCP role for all care. Often the PCP steps aside in favor of the specialist, who addresses only a particular bodily system. As a result a Status One patient has no clinician assuming responsibility for overall clinical care and social-support needs.

Access to Care

Status One patients should have regularly scheduled PCP appointments. The clinical record may reveal long waits for access to the PCP, specialists, or diagnostic testing. Transportation or child-care barriers are mentioned at times or may be revealed by direct discussion with the patient. The more unstable patients may require twenty-four-hour phone access to a knowledgeable person who can answer their questions.

Process of Care

The care process for patients seen episodically in the ER, in urgent care, or as inpatients is probably uncoordinated. Similarly, repetitive tests, care deviating significantly from appropriate guidelines, repeat visits for the same complaint without resolution or a plan, and unaddressed opportunities for home care may indicate a process of care not serving the patient's needs.

Coordination of Care

The comprehensive medical care review may reveal important gaps in coordination. There may be no clinical care plan, no integration of the care provided by numerous clinicians, uncoordinated treatments in which dosing titration is important (for example, insulin injections or Coumadin anticoagulation), or no advanced directives specifying the type of care for life-threatening emergencies.

Documentation of Care

Documenting care is important when many providers are involved or unplanned ER visits and hospital admissions are likely. In the absence of good information in an emergency, the health care system will automatically default to the highest acuity care, with associated high expense. Documentation often missing or incomplete includes problem lists, medication lists, the current plan of care, or a discharge summary from a recent hospitalization.

Patient Involvement

The medical care review may reveal that information is not shared by providers and patients. Patient inquiries may remain unanswered; opportunities for involvement or patient education may have been missed; pharmacists may not have been involved despite a complex drug regimen; or the patient may not have been told how to contact clinicians for urgent care or emergency triage.

Follow-Up

Even the best clinical plans will be ineffective unless there is follow-up. The medical review sometimes shows that abnormal laboratory results, ER and urgent-care episodes, or the care plans themselves have not been communicated or acted on.

• • • • • • •

This chapter covered practices surrounding the assessment of Status One patients. New patients are first identified to the care manager through predictive algorithms supplemented by clinical judgment. Every Status One patient is assigned a dedicated care manager who is responsible for performing the assessment and later for devising the care plan. Assessments are based on direct client contact and questionnaires. The process includes identifying what is important to the client and the client's goals. A comprehensive medical review examines clinical care for gaps and omissions.

. . . .

6

Formulating Care Plans
To Each According to Their Needs

High-risk population health management is a systematic approach to assessing both the coordination of medical care and a variety of social factors. An operational model integrating psychological and social factors with medical care creates the framework for assessment and care planning used by care managers to enable Status One patients to improve their quality of life and to require less costly medical care. This chapter describes the model and the six aims of managing high-risk patients, five of which complement the traditional coordination of medical care.

Up to this point, we have seen that a managed care population can be stratified by risk of future clinical complexities and cost. Existing electronically accessible databases can be employed to point to these people. Care managers form a long-term relationship with the patient, beginning with the assessment process as a prelude to customized health action plans.

Current Narrow Focus on Clinical Issues

When physicians and nurses interact with Status One patients, they naturally gravitate to the content of clinical care. It is an area in which they feel comfortable. The complexity of the patient's situation and the time constraints imposed by clinical practice and

health planning typically work together to promote a strictly clinical view. The average PCP, seeing such a patient during a ten- or
fifteen-minute appointment, has little choice.

Opportunities to improve functional status and reduce the need
for near-term high-intensity services often come from outside the
narrowly defined clinical realm. When challenged to describe the
frail and chronically ill patients for whom they did the most good,
focus groups of clinicians that we led preceding the first Status One
program gave instances of uncovering and addressing important
social and psychological aspects of the cases. Such opportunities
existed across broad diagnostic categories, ages, and social back-
grounds. Decreased future needs for costly care resulted more from
addressing the psychosocial issues than from discovering glaring gaps
in clinical care.

During traditional medical residency training, physicians have
been taught to call for the social worker when encountering the
chronically ill and complex patient, in situations where these
aspects are considered important. At such a juncture, they conclude
that their clinical work is done. Little changes over the years. The
approach is not confined to doctors. In fact, nurse case managers
still declare, "I didn't go to nursing school to become a social
worker." The problem posed by this attitude is that episodic clinical interventions arising out of ambulatory and inpatient care of any
kind—medical, nursing, or social work—rarely have a lasting effect
on the future course of Status One patients.

At times clinicians are concerned exclusively with the coordination of medical care, and they ignore or rationalize disengage-
ment with psychological and social issues. For too many health
professionals, labeling a patient as having complex psychosocial
issues seems tantamount to abdicating their ability to influence the
broader social-support system in these patients' lives.

Medical social work arguably has the best grasp of this area,
although there are strong conceptual frameworks in family medicine (Noble, 1997) and the core nursing process (Smeltzer,

Suddarth, and Bare, 1996). Unfortunately, current incentives encourage no one to use, develop, or refine such approaches.

Case Example 6.1. Missed Social Issues as a Factor in High Health Care Utilization

Claire Eisen is a seventy-three-year-old woman who suffered a femoral neck fracture, a kind of hip fracture that is unfortunately common in elderly women with osteoporotic weak bones. The woman had other diagnoses, none serious in themselves, but they interacted with each other to limit her functional status. These conditions included mild cataracts and hypertension. She was a member of a Medicare HMO.

A resident's admission history prior to orthopedic surgery revealed that Ms. Eisen earnestly desired to travel to Texas to visit her only daughter and her family at Christmas. She was concerned that her medical conditions would limit her ability to make the visit.

An internal pinning and fixation procedure proceeded without operative complications. After a brief inpatient course of rehabilitation, Ms. Eisen was discharged with home-care rehabilitation services for several weeks. When she reached a plateau of ambulation with the aid of a free-standing walker, further care was discontinued.

Case managers were focused on rapid completion of the episode of clinical care, citing inpatient length-of-stay guidelines for the femoral-fracture Disease Related Group and sparing use of rehabilitation services. No care provider took the time to understand Ms. Eisen's real motivation nor worked to help her attain her goal. Rather, standard guidelines, algorithms, criteria, expectations, and missed opportunities prevailed.

Unused to her newly limited walking ability, she missed appointments for controlling her blood pressure and was reluctant to undertake surgical correction of her cataracts. She did not know who could help her with travel tips and assistance. She never did visit her daughter at Christmas.

She stayed close to home, becoming more isolated and depressed from her diminished functionality. Within a year she suffered a stroke whose hemiparesis combined with her social isolation to propel her toward institutionalization. As clinicians review her care, they might see the outcome as inevitable and overlook the underlying causes and missed opportunities.

Although Ms. Eisen was a Status One patient, assessment and planning did not address what was truly important to her. Instead, it focused on the immediate clinical situation. One is left to wonder whether the complications would have occurred with the same severity and high cost if care management had properly assessed the important family and social motivations and enabled Ms. Eisen to access additional care and to achieve her goals.

One thing is certain: the Medicare HMO paid the full costs for all of Ms. Eisen's care, and these costs amounted to many times the premiums paid on her behalf.

Psychosocial Contributors to High Utilization

Evidence is beginning to accumulate about the importance of subclinical depression, isolation, and a variety of social challenges as modifiable risk factors for high-cost care. A randomized, controlled study in Washington State (Leveille and others, 1998) tracked hospital use in the year following enrollment of chronically ill, community-dwelling seniors in an activity and support group; they were matched with controls who pursued their usual activities. Subsequent inpatient days were reduced 71 percent in the experimental group, and hospital admissions were reduced 38 percent. Two remarkable aspects of this study were the extent to which people with chronic illnesses could be empowered to achieve their goals and self-sufficiency and the extent to which this approach dramatically reduced demand for and use of expensive medical services. The conjoined social and clinical approach evident in the Leveille work is explicitly incorporated into the care of Status One patients. There is every reason to believe that such dynamics apply to younger adults in commercial HMOs, people for whom community resources are scarce compared with those available to seniors.

Other studies show the influence of social isolation and depressive symptoms on adverse outcomes in such common and morbid conditions as cerebral vascular accidents (Morris and others, 1993), myocardial infarctions (Frasure-Smith and others, 1993), and femoral fractures (Mossey and others, 1990).

Breaking the Noncompliance Conundrum

A common and unproductive dynamic deserves to be singled out so that it can be avoided. Health professionals believe they know best what patients or clients need for their health conditions. Whether or not the person agrees, prescribed actions become the basis of a traditional care plan. The action plan is "doing it to them," often casting clients in a passive role and constricting their own ability to influence the situation (Snyder, 1994). When clients do not follow through on the plan, they are labeled as noncompliant.

The noncompliant client in today's health care system is considered to be in need of "education." Even worse, health professionals may discount these individuals for further attention once they did not do as they are told. Nevertheless, the noncompliant client is still at risk for further problems (Eraker, 1984). In managed care, this risk is also financial for the MCO or risk-bearing delivery system. Something must change.

Status One health action plans are pursued in a client-centered fashion. Actions are based on aims revealed by the assessment process to be important to the client. Actions are part of a contract made with the client. Clinicians focus on the client's priorities and look for opportunities over time to introduce new issues that they see as important.

Theoretical Underpinnings of Status One Aims

Status One patients benefit from a systematic application of models of human motivation and also of ideas about an individual's "circle of influence."

Theories of Human Motivation

Maslow (1943) proposed these human motivations:

1. Basic physiological needs: hunger, thirst, sex
2. Safety needs: protection from physical sources of harm, shelter from the weather
3. Belonging and affiliation needs: liking oneself, affection, care and support
4. Esteem needs: respect, positive regard, status, recognition
5. Self-actualization needs: fulfillment of one's potential

At the base of a pyramid of drives rests the need to fulfill innate metabolic drives. Breathing and eating are requisite to life and quickly extinguish life if denied. Sexual activity is similarly programmed into human neurophysiology and anatomy, and is viewed as a basal need in Maslow's scheme. Only slightly less immediate is the quest for safety, whether it be protection from heat, cold, and the extremes of the elements or from physical dangers posed by external forces. Aside from needs to preserve the individual, humans seek the company of others, along with the positive feelings of affiliation, esteem, and respect that can come only from interaction with other people. The highest state of being is self-actualization, the individual's quest and attainment of his or her full potential. Maslow presented his five motivations as a hierarchy because he thought little could be accomplished toward fulfilling higher order goals if more basic needs went unfulfilled.

The concept has strong intuitive appeal, especially in extreme and acute cases. It would be hard to conceive of someone giving much thought to earning the esteem and good will of colleagues while being unable to fend off starvation. In the workplace, Maslow observed that those in excessively hazardous occupations and those not earning enough money for food and shelter are motivated to strike or to join aggressive unions. Well-paid employees have different, more abstract goals, beyond physiologic and safety requirements.

Despite widespread recognition of Maslow's hierarchy and its continued application in a number of fields, since its introduction more than fifty years ago it has found little support in the research on organizational behavior (Wahba and Bridwell, 1976).

More recently Alderfer (1969) proposed three areas of human needs:

1. Existence: hunger, thirst, protection
2. Relatedness: social and affiliation needs, regard
3. Growth: realization of one's potential

He based his views on detailed questionnaires covering the needs, wants, and aspirations of all the employees working for a bank. "Existence" is similar to Maslow's first and second hierarchical levels—those bearing on the most basic physiological needs and on individual physical safety. "Relatedness" captures Maslow's needs for both affiliation and positive esteem. "Growth" is close conceptually to Maslow's self-actualization.

Alderfer is less rigid than Maslow in insisting that one level must be satisfied before progressing to the next. Rather than asserting a satisfaction and progression sequence, Alderfer contended that the motivation to address an area is highest when that need is at an extreme. The impetus to modify one of Alderfer's aspects of human motivation is more related to its being either very satisfied or very unsatisfied rather than to the extent to which lower aims on the hierarchy have been addressed. Psychological and organizational-behavior research has been supportive of such classifiable themes in human activities and aspirations (Wanous and Zwany, 1977).

A relatively new concept is the assertion that higher order motivators exist in the face of chronic illness (Lorig and others, 1994). Affiliation and higher purpose may be even more important to the chronically ill than they are to the healthy. Thwarting them can markedly contribute to rapidly decreasing functional status and eventually to high-acuity and costly medical care. Conversely, actively engaging Status One patients on this level yields dramatic near-term results in economic and functional status.

Five of the six Status One aims (described below) tease out components of "psychosocial" issues. Two themes are interwoven: individual responsibility and the client/patient as part of a social network.

Circle of Influence and Circle of Concern

A new concept of what modulates an individual's level of influence and effectiveness at the individual, group, and family level has emerged (Covey, 1989). Put forth as an attribute of effective leaders, it is also useful in visualizing Status One patient needs. Those aspects of life under a person's immediate control constitute the Circle of Influence, as shown in the circle on the left in Figure 6.1. Factors outside may be of great interest, but the individual cannot directly influence or change them. Effective leaders focus their energies in the Circle of Influence. Over time, they have a positive impact and make changes. The Circle of Influence enlarges as others recognize results and the individual has an opportunity to tackle more issues and projects (illustrated by the circle on the right in Figure 6.1). People who spend their time in the Circle of Concern accomplish nothing. Over time, their influence decreases as does their personal power and energy.

In the clinical arena the many challenges of illness and injury narrow the patient's perceived Circle of Influence (Figure 6.2). The

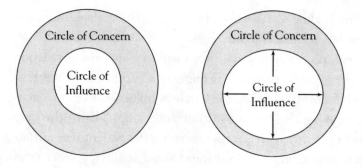

Figure 6.1. Circle of Influence and Circle of Concern. Positive energy enlarges the Circle of Influence.

Source: Adapted from S. R. Covey, *The Seven Basic Habits of Highly Effective People.* By permission.

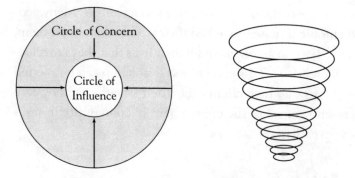

Figure 6.2. Effect of Chronic Illness on the Circle of Influence. A downward spiral of isolation, depression, and lowered functionality ends in a worsening clinical state.

Source: Adapted from S. R. Covey, *The Seven Basic Habits of Highly Effective People.* By permission.

health establishment's response is to provide clinical services, to do things for the patient, without encouraging what the patient is able to do. The term *patient* and the structure of the inpatient model reinforce the person as a passive recipient of care. The unintended result is to further narrow patients' perceived Circle of Influence and to widen the Circle of Concern until patients with a chronic debilitating condition feel they have little or no influence over their own lives. All too often the result is to stifle higher order aspirations and plans, leading to a downward cycle of isolation, depression, and growing dependence on costly, high-acuity medical care.

A key aspect of care management within a high-risk population health management strategy is to engage the patient in any way possible to refocus attention on the Circle of Influence, even in a matter like having the patient initiate follow-up calls to the care manager rather than vice versa (assuming the patient sees initiating such calls as an important step toward achieving short-term goals). Modest steps toward self-care and autonomy enlarge the Circle of Influence and can break the downward spiral of increasing dependence on the health care system.

Several of the Status One aims include self-reliance and the interdependence of the patient within a social context. Many people with chronic illnesses have had their worlds close in on them, or they have been so autonomous all their lives that they are reluctant to call on others. This cycle of social isolation can be averted with care plans that help clients map their situation and by care managers who empower the engagement of community in ways important to patients.

Aims for Managing Status One Patients

The six aims for managing Status One patients (Exhibit 6.1) are based on current best practices in managing high-risk patients. They provide an orderly foundation for assessing patient situations and

1. Coordination of medical care
2. Self-reliance
3. Daily activity and fitness
4. Interdependence with family and friends
5. Mental challenge
6. Community involvement and purpose

Exhibit 6.1. Six Aims for Status One Patients.

building effective care plans. They rationalize the processes of care management and are associated with breakthrough economic and functional outcomes for a most challenging group of patients. The aims also provide a promising arena for further research into the dynamics and intervention opportunities for the care of at-risk subpopulations.

Aim 1: Coordination of Medical Care

Coordinating medical care is the more traditional arena of clinical care and case management. Aspects include arranging for and authorizing the involvement of appropriate clinicians, access to care, care processes, coordination and documentation of care, patient involvement, and follow-up. Chapter Five discussed these aspects in detail.

Aim 2: Self-Reliance

In the patient-centered approach, patients actively participate in and assume responsibility for their care. The clinical condition may preclude full self-sufficiency and self-management, but even modest increases in self-reliance, as evidenced in concrete behaviors that are part of a contract with Status One patients, can have a significant positive impact. Existing case management approaches all too often foster passivity by providing services and indirectly reinforcing a growing dependence on the health care system.

Aim 3: Daily Activity and Fitness

Movement and activity can be important at any age. Although the term *fitness* may conjure up visions of health clubs and youthful, muscular physiques, simple movements and mobility strengthen self-reliance in addition to providing intrinsic benefits. In our experience, any increase in the level of activity, perhaps as modest as having a homebound patient walk to fetch the mail once a day, has a disproportionately positive impact on a patient's well-being.

Aim 4: Interdependence with Family and Friends

The patients and their social networks are interdependent and dynamic. If the network is strong, the health action plan will incorporate the participation of family and friends. The weakness or absence of a network needs to be recognized and addressed if such a group is critical to the patient and the care plan.

A frequent trap is to substitute the health delivery system for a real or potential community. In Meals on Wheels programs, for example, the nutritional supplementation is often not as important as the daily social contact for shut-ins. It is preferable to rely on family and friends to supply services of low clinical content rather than to have home-care or other high-intensity services supply them.

Aim 5: Mental Challenge

Interest in surroundings, hobbies, reading, and other passions stimulates the mind. Status One patients who surrender their interests and stimulating thoughts tend to focus on their clinical woes.

Aim 6: Community Involvement and Sense of Purpose

Isolation from the community and loss of higher purpose can be both a result of health challenges and an opportunity to further magnify ills and isolation. With terminal illnesses, the focus needs to be on life's meaning, spirituality, and the closing of affairs; facilitating this focus may take the intervention of a care manager. The absence or constriction of community involvement and aspirations to higher purpose, especially when they had been important motivators to an individual, contributes to lowering functional status and increasing the likelihood of costly, high-acuity care.

Steps in Formulating the Health Action Plan

Action plans are the shared responsibility of the client and the care manager. Client participation is the hallmark of effective care planning. The care manager's responsibility is to integrate the client and clinical perspectives in order to formulate goals, aims, and actions.

Researching and Identifying Possible Actions

Formulating a health action plan begins with researching and identifying potential health actions. The novice care manager can start by identifying one to three actions for each Status One aim the client considers important. Health actions are designed to achieve incremental change from the starting point rather than an optimal state.

In addition to the health assessment questionnaire and comprehensive medical review, additional tools support development and execution of health action plans. These tools can be augmented by automated care plan software, especially those that are intranet-based. As explained in Chapter Three, secure intranets enable access to the care plan from any location, and they also provide links to reference sites, guidelines, experts, and community resources. The internet also provides a foundation for patient involvement because of its direct connection into the home.

Consultations with experts on a variety of issues that can be barriers to individual care planning are a useful tool for care managers. These e-mail advisors are providing a high-technology equivalent of "curbside consults"—the practice of accosting colleagues for advice on difficult cases. The breadth of possible situations encountered with Status One patients makes this an essential functionality. Status One plans work best when experts have been incorporated into the process.

Such consultations are not meant to substitute for specialty clinical visits, but rather to obtain authoritative input in puzzling situations. The consultant typically will not know the patient's name. Topics in frequent demand include such ancillary and nonmedical issues as health care proxy, housing, and respite care.

E-mail arrangements through an intranet widen the circle of these consultations to anyone in the institution or in the community who has clearance and has agreed to support care planning. Exhibit C is a form that can be used by the care management lead team to identify advice topics and experts for loading into online reference files. Exhibit D is the Status One consultant's role description. Exhibit E is a sample letter to a new consultant, describing the consultant's role in advising care managers in an area of expertise. Exhibit F is a form that can be used to record information on each consultant.

Resource directories include community and institutional services that may be enlisted in the care planning process. Like consultations, they work best when identified and screened in advance. Current approaches all too often leave a case manager to hunt for needed services in the course of developing a care plan, a wholly unsatisfactory way to deal with at-risk Status One clients.

Clinical guidelines are rarely useful in their entirety because of Status One clients' comorbidities and other complexities. Nevertheless, portions of guidelines can be useful as a touchstone for some aspects of care. They should be readily available to the care manager at the time the plan is being formulated.

On the internet *hot links* allow access to web sites that can provide anything from names of local community support groups to authoritative references on obscure diseases from national advocacy groups to the National Library of Medicine. Suitably designed intranet applications enable the care manager to go freely from the health action plan to a variety of supportive internet sites and back again.

Integrating the Client's Goals

The most fruitful part of care planning is aligning key goals, aims, and actions with the client. Prior to meeting with the client, it is important to conceive an approach. Differences between clinical priorities and those of the client are addressed over time. Consultation with the PCP or specialist to gain understanding of the patient's situation and to secure suggestions about the plan is essential.

It is helpful to write down potential actions to discuss with the client at the first meeting (see Exhibit G). At this time an important bond is formed between the patient and care manager that will serve as the basis for the relationship. Expect the meeting with the client (and the family, if appropriate) to last thirty to forty-five minutes. Begin with introductions, a review of the health assessment questionnaire, and agreement on key aims. Let the client talk; this discussion is not about what the care manager can do for the client but what the client can do for himself or herself. Outputs include a health action plan signed by the client and care manager, the client's genuine commitment to follow through on incremental steps, and a follow-up appointment.

Involving Physicians

PCPs will vary widely in their involvement with Status One health action planning. The process accommodates a range of participation from passive concurrence to active, close collaboration with the care manager. Most often physicians welcome additional attention to their problematic clients, and occasionally they provide detailed input. Many care managers find it useful to schedule regular time with the PCP to discuss Status One issues at one time, regardless of where the patients are in the care planning process.

No physician will have more than a handful of Status One patients at any time. In our experience geriatricians with full managed care panels have the most Status One patients, as many as twenty at a time. The mean for PCP internists is four to six.

Using Ideas About the Stages of Change

Once the care manager and client have determined specific health issues or problems needing modification and chosen and prioritized the behaviors the client is willing to change, they need to establish realistic steps toward reaching behavioral goals. Prochaska's model for stages of change (Prochaska, Norcross, and DiClemente, 1994) is particularly useful in gauging clients' readiness and appropriate actions for them.

In the *precontemplation* stage, the client is not seriously considering changing a behavior or lifestyle or is not considering alternatives to working with permanent limitations. An effective strategy for the care manager is to raise awareness of risks and limitations, provide personalized information, identify the benefits of change, assist in expressing and dealing with emotional issues, and indicate a readiness to help when the client is ready to make a change.

In the *contemplation* stage, clients are ready to accept the challenge posed by the problem or limitation. They may be seriously thinking about changing their lifestyle or considering new alternatives in the near term. They do not yet have a plan of action. The care manager's strategy should be to increase clients' confidence in their ability to change, assist in clarifying values, address barriers to change, offer a wide array of alternatives, and reduce ambivalence.

In the *preparation* stage, the client is intending to take action in the next month, may have unsuccessfully taken actions already in the past year, and may report small lifestyle changes. The care manager's strategy is to help resolve ambivalence, develop and encourage commitment to an action plan, break down the behavior or lifestyle change into manageable steps, and identify and reward any small changes that have been made.

The *action* phase is where care managers and providers hope their Status One clients will be, but experience indicates that as few as a quarter will be at this point at the initiation of the health action plan. In this stage clients are in the process of modifying behavior, experiences, and environment to cope with the challenges, problems, or limitations to their lifestyle. The care manager's strategies should include negotiating short-term goals, identifying needed supports, substituting alternatives for problem behaviors, suggesting how to avoid relapse to the old lifestyle and how to overcome barriers, rewarding positive changes, and identifying follow-up actions.

In *maintenance* the client has been pursuing the activities of the action stage for six or more months. The care manager's task is to prevent the client from relapsing to the old lifestyle. Care manager strategies include suggesting how to meet new challenges and overcome new limitations, identifying family or local resources and supports, problem solving, identifying a strategy to deal with relapse, and continuing to recognize positive changes.

In the *relapse* stage clients have fallen back to previous behaviors and accepted limitations. They may be demoralized; they feel that they have failed and may want to give up. The care manager can play a positive role by identifying the cause of the relapse, working with the client on a plan for getting back on track, and reminding the client that many people who have been successful with their plans have tried more than once.

Case Example 6.2. Determining Stage of Change

Mary Benner, who has multiple chronic illnesses, has been widowed for two years. Since her husband's death she has significantly reduced her attendance at social events and has cut down her contacts with friends and neighbors. Her illnesses are becoming more acute, and her condition is deteriorating. When her husband was alive, they were a socially active couple. Ms. Benner tells you that she misses the contact and wishes that she could gradually increase her social activities.

Ms. Benner is in the preparation stage of behavior change. Here, the care manager plays the most positive role by laying out various alternatives that meet Ms. Benner's aim of community involvement and by negotiating with Ms. Benner specific actions that will bring her toward her goal.

Negotiating Patient Contracts

A process of negotiating contracts with people who have chronic diseases has been developed by Lorig (Lorig and others, 1994). We have found it to be a powerful concept when applied to Status One clients.

To break the noncompliance conundrum, it is important that health actions be something that the client wants to do and has truly agreed to do. These may be actions they have committed themselves to do, such as calling the care manager for a weekly follow-up, or actions that the health system will do, such as arranging for transportation for a key specialist consultation. The action must be reasonable and specific, and must answer the questions "what, how much, when, how often."

If there is doubt about clients' commitment, asking them to rate their confidence that they will follow through on a scale of 1 to 10 can be helpful. Scores of 7 or higher indicate that the client is likely to follow through.

Coordinating Interventions

During this phase the care manager coordinates and communicates required interventions to all responsible parties, including the client. A work scheduler that specifies client needs and responsibilities is necessary for a care manager tracking numerous health actions for a panel of Status One patients.

* * * * * * *

In this chapter the six aims of Status One care planning were introduced: coordinated medical care, self-reliance, daily activity and fitness, interdependence with family and friends, mental challenge, and community involvement and a sense of purpose. The challenge posed by the noncompliant patient was discussed, as was an effective approach maximizing patient autonomy, recognizing readiness to change, and specifying actions in the care plan.

Renewals and Endings
Reassessment and Discharge

U p to this point, the process of improving care for the highest-risk managed care members, the Status One patients, has been taken from systematic identification through assessment and care planning. This process amalgamates clinical and social approaches.

Reassessment

The next part of the process, reassessment, involves coordination and shared responsibility with the client. Here, care managers integrate client and clinical perspectives to update goals, aims, and health actions. They identify successes and failures, revise goals and aims, reformulate health action plans, and renegotiate actions with the client.

Recall from Chapter Five that acuity levels are a means of incorporating professional judgment into care planning. They permit a care manager to triage patients already identified as high risk. Acuity level 1 indicates a judgment that hospitalization or other high-intensity medical care is likely in the next three months, while acuity level 5 signifies a judgment that the need for such care is more than two years away. Combining the predictive algorithms that identify Status One patients with the care manager's and PCP's judgment, as captured in the acuity level, makes a clinical registry useful and continually refocused on those people most in need.

Acuity levels are set according to the best available information at the time and should be reset as necessary during reassessment.

Reassessment includes an updating not only of acuity but also of functional status. For these purposes we recommend using the patients' global summary of their health rather than a more comprehensive screening instrument such as the SF-36 (Ware, Snow, Kosinski, and Gandek, 1995). The reassessment also includes a reexamination of the medical record and a discussion of the patient's progress with key physicians prior to meeting with the patient.

Frequency

Reassessment of the patient's situation and the care plan should be done every six to eight weeks for the most unstable clients, those judged by the care manager to be at acuity levels 1 and 2. As acuity improves, reassessments can be less frequent. An important clinical behavioral change that the client did not agree to in an earlier action plan should be revisited at reassessment if the client's readiness for such a change has increased. Gratifying changes are often realized after subsequent care plan updates, especially with people who might otherwise have been written off as noncompliant.

Status One members with an acuity level of 3 or 4 may be reassessed at intervals of eight to twelve weeks. For acuity level 5, the follow-up could be as simple as ascertaining that prescribed medication is being taken and scheduling routine follow-up care with the PCP. An acute event expected to change the content and direction of the care plan—for example, a new hospitalization, a stroke, or a new myocardial infarction—always triggers a reassessment in order to modify the care plan to fit the new circumstances.

Principles Underlying Reassessment

Empirically, several tactics combine to produce the most effective care plans. The care management nurse and client together update changed portions of the functional health assessment. Encouragement and praise are given liberally for current healthy behaviors. The belief is expressed that the client is capable of making necessary changes. If they have failed to implement agreed-on behaviors, the stages of the change model described in the previous chapter should be reviewed. Rather than apply the noncompliant label, the care manager should revise the care plan with the client to reflect the client's problem-solving efforts and to outline a new approach for implementing behavior changes and meeting goals.

Discharge

Clients no longer at risk for intensive, high-cost medical care within the next twelve months may be discharged from the Status One registry to a less proactive disease management program or to primary care. In the population-based approach to health management, the discharge of Status One patients has a distinct set of implications. Patients eligible for discharge may be at lower risk for clinical complications and high costs than when they were first identified and placed on the Status One registry. However, discharge does not mean that they will not have complications, but rather that the risk has been lessened and that the situation overall is stable.

From a data-management perspective discharge means that predictive algorithms no longer detect the patterns of care that suggest high risk. In our experience, the predictive models are set to examine data from as far back as the previous twelve months. As the twelve-month window advances month by month, the sentinel situations may fall out from the window for those patients who are stabilizing.

Discharge from Status One is not the same as a cure. Such patients often have more than one condition simultaneously in addition to frequent social-support and subclinical psychological issues. Clinically, a cure may not be expected and is rarely achieved.

Discharge may be precipitated by insurance changes. Independent of any change in the clinical situation, the member may switch to a different health plan or provider group or may simply move out of the area. In risk-bearing provider groups, there will be no adverse impact on the patient if the insurance change is from one globally capitated plan to another. A more difficult situation arises with a change from managed care to a fee-for-service plan—for example, a change from a Medicare risk product to traditional Medicare reimbursements. The clinicians will be the same in this case. Each group must determine how it will approach such situations, which are fortunately rare. Financial incentives are better aligned with intensive care management for Status One patients within managed care than for those under fee for service. When the care managers are hired by an insurer, a change in insurance plan leads directly to a discharge decision.

Criteria for Discharge

Properly done, care planning for high-risk patients should be a smooth transition over time rather than an abrupt change. Status One clients who have made progress toward their goals should already have had significant time following their plan, thereby increasing self-reliant actions and lowering their acuity level. They should be in a position to benefit from a lower, appropriate level of care. Their dependence on the care manager should now be much less than it was when they began.

Criteria for deciding on discharge from care management include progress in achieving goals, a lowered risk of future high resource utilization, and a judgment that the health action plan is no longer required to keep the risk low. Administrative changes described above may also lead to a discharge decision.

Detours on the Road to Discharge

Care managers and clinicians may follow several unproductive practices without the guidance of leaders. If patient care plans have fostered dependence on the health care system, it will be difficult to wean patients from them. In unstable situations continued care is amply justified, but in many other instances the lonely and isolated have not established a social-support network of friends, family, and the community but instead have come to depend for nonclinical support on health care providers. Such situations frequently arise with home-care nurses and home health aides.

PCPs or care managers can have difficulty letting go. The appreciative patient, the pleasant patient, the greatly improved patient are people with whom professionals like to work. In the Status One group, where the overall prognosis is fair at best, it is natural for nurses, doctors, and social workers to want to hold on to successes and patients who give them positive feedback.

Changed eligibility can cause plans to go awry. An active care plan on which a former member's health depends must have a smooth transition, rather than being withdrawn suddenly.

The net impact of too many detours on the road to discharge is a traffic jam. New Status One patients are added to the registry at a rate of 10 to 15 percent a month. If many patients are retained who no longer are in the highest-risk category, the attention of care managers will be diverted from the new, as yet unassessed, Status One patients to relatively better patients who have been on the registry for some time.

On Track for Discharge

Status One patients are on track toward discharge when the six aims are achieved as far as possible and coordination of medical care is good; they are no longer judged as being at high risk for hospitalization and high costs within the upcoming year. Other reassuring developments are that major barriers to the best feasible health condition are no longer present, the patient is positively involved and empowered, and a structure and plan for ongoing care are in place.

Required Discharge Actions

Performing certain actions ensures that discharge proceeds smoothly. Ongoing clinical care is assured by scheduling a follow-up appointment with the PCP. The patient knows whom to contact for "slippage" from maintenance and when to do so. This contact person can be the care manager or the PCP's office.

Closure with the client is important for the care manager. Closure may come from a simple statement such as, "Dr. Jones and I have been happy to support you over the past year as you have worked to improve your situation. I no longer need to follow you as closely as before." A brief notation in the care plan documents the interaction and can be useful if conditions should worsen in the future.

It is possible that the patient will return to the Status One registry. Paper copies of the assessment tools, including the comprehensive medical review, are retained for possible future use. If the patient returns to the Status One level, the assessment process can be shortened by updating the previously collected data.

Elective Retention as Status One

If the care manager and PCP judge that certain patients are still at high risk despite their imminent departure from the Status One registry, they can selectively retain those people in an active care plan. Patients whose acuity level remains at 1 to 3 are automatically candidates for retention. Provider or care manager intuition and concern can be a powerful tool when used in this way.

Case Example 7.1. Nonretention of a Status One Patient

After twelve months on the registry, a congestive heart failure (CHF) patient is following a care plan based on daily weight charts, the addition of angiotensin converting enzyme inhibitor medication, weekly visits by a volunteer, and weekly calls to the care manager. Additional clinical conditions include glaucoma and eczema, both controlled with medications.

Should the patient be discharged from intensive-care management?

Yes. If reassessments have revealed that the plan is being carried out well, the client may be returned to ordinary ambulatory care. At the time of discharge, the care manager makes sure that the client has scheduled clinical follow-up and knows the appropriate point of contact should the situation worsen in the future. If the organization has a CHF disease management program, enrolling the client in it is an alternative. Assessments and the comprehensive medical care review are retained in case they are needed in the future.

. . . .

Case Example 7.2. Retention of a Status One Patient

A diabetic who tends to have foot and calf infections has been followed for twelve months. He has made no headway on actions supporting his aims. His blood HbA$_1$c is 12.1, higher than before. Social isolation and physical inactivity continue unabated.

Should the patient be discharged from intensive care management?

No. Retain the poorly controlled diabetic under care management. It is likely that the predictive models would continue to retain him automatically. If they did not, the patient is a candidate for provider-designated retention. The situation should be reassessed and an updated health action plan developed with the patient.

. . . .

Case Example 7.3. Limited Retention of a Status One Patient

After five months as a Status One patient, an eighty-year-old woman who has osteoporosis and had a post-fall hip replacement has met her goals. These include participating in an arts program at the local senior day-care center, improvement of home safety, and a medication review.

Should the patient be discharged from intensive care management?

Yes. The predictive model will retain her on the registry automatically until after the factors that triggered her registry listing have passed. Since she is doing quite well, her acuity level may be downgraded to 4 or 5. The care plan may be reduced to minimal actions that provide positive feedback and that help the woman hold her gains. Monitoring by phone monthly until discharge would be an adequate plan in these circumstances.

· · · · · · ·

In this chapter the rationale and mechanics of reassessments and care plan renewals were explained. When Status One patients no longer meet the highest risk level as identified by the computer algorithms, they may be discharged to a lower appropriate level of care. Alternatively, they may be retained selectively by the care manager and PCP.

. . . .

8

Gauges on the Dashboard
Process and Outcome Measures

This chapter lays out an essential set of measures for high-risk population health management. Emphasis and examples are based on systematic management of the highest-risk group, the Status One patients. The first three chapters discussed the rationale and mechanics for stratifying a managed care population into groups based on predicted future clinical needs. Succeeding chapters described clinical registries of high-risk patients, assessment methods, care planning for individual patients, and reassessments and discharge of patients from the Status One registry.

Essential Metrics

A minimal set of metrics is necessary to monitor and direct effort toward the Status One patients on the high-risk registry and to gauge aggregate costs, utilization rates, and process outcomes. Based on the needs of clinical and administrative leaders, the population metrics are most often subsets of financial and utilization measures of their overall membership's experience.

Financial and utilization metrics have traditionally focused on cost per member per month (PMPM) and hospital utilization per one thousand members. A process includes the steps, activities, and interactions that bring about a desired result. Process outcomes reflect the result of the sum of these activities. Good process

measures isolate the important activities so that they point to contributions toward the end result and provide a yardstick for
improvements.

What to Measure

For Status One patient care it is well to keep in mind how the registry of highest-risk patients is defined so that the chosen metrics
reflect the relevant experience. The Status One registry results from
a computerized model of predictive patterns of care consistently
applied each month to data from the previous twelve-month window. The Status One registry, like other disease registries from a
population, is a snapshot of all the members meeting inclusion criteria in that month.

Metrics reflect the cost data, utilization rates, and basic well-
being of all members in the Status One registry in the month. Some
measurements relate to important aspects of the process of providing
care; others are results and outcomes of such care. The epidemiological concept employed is called cross-sectional prevalence, which
is explained further in Chapter Fourteen. Importantly, though, these
metrics are not based on a static cohort of patients over time, but
rather on the experience of anyone identified within the registry at
any given time.

There are deliberate omissions from Status One metrics. Patients
who are added on the intuition of care managers or PCPs are not
included because criteria for invoking such judgments differ widely.
Some clinicians are enthusiastic, early adopters of Status One care
management and are liberal in the inclusion of additional patients
not identified by the computerized algorithm. Other providers support the care planning process only for those identified by computer
modeling. Some patients are electively continued in care planning
despite their improving sufficiently to no longer trip the computerized algorithms identifying high risk. Added patients of all types,
who swell the Status One registry 5 to 15 percent on the average,
receive the full benefit of care management and planning.

The aggregate metrics, which do not include added patients, reflect experience consistently across providers and locations. However, metrics for the patients added by clinicians can be evaluated on an ad hoc basis separately from those produced regularly for ongoing research.

Month-to-Month Variation

With the diversity of diseases, comorbidities, and social situations of Status One patients, month-to-month variation in the results is expected. The variation is particularly great when the size of the Status One group drops below several hundred. Trends over time are more meaningful than a change one way or the other over a few months. In order to construct a performance trend line, historical monthly statistics for the prior year can be run retrospectively. This retrospective assessment establishes a valid baseline and discerns any temporal trends that may already be present.

Upper and lower control limits can also be established on the trend of monthly data points. It takes at least twelve monthly data points to establish such limits and the same amount of time to average out seasonal variation in the incidence of illnesses. Medical leaders can establish baseline and control limits for Status One (or for any subpopulation) measures by retroactively establishing the prior year's experience from historical data.

Financial and Utilization Measures

Statistical models that stratify a subpopulation based on administrative data can and should produce PMPM cost and hospital admissions metrics for this membership group. Surprisingly, many MCOs do not have such fundamental information at hand. Those that do may have it only for a single payer or insurance product line or in a form adulterated by variable application of expenses that were incurred but not recorded (called IBNR by accountants and actuaries). Although it is recommended that the most recent data, even if incomplete, be used to produce patient registries for clinical use, financial and utilization data can not be gathered for several months, until claims are paid. Use of IBNR can be avoided if cost metrics are produced once claims are essentially complete (after approximately ninety to one hundred twenty days). IBNR estimations can deviate greatly and unpredictably from actual experience.

Overall PMPM cost is the actual monthly expenses for the entire membership expressed on the basis of an average per member. PMPM cost is one of the chief endpoints of a managed care organization. It is a measure of economic efficiency in the rendering of health care. Overall PMPM cost is calculated by dividing total actual expenses for all care by member-months.

Status One PMPM cost is the actual costs incurred for Status One patients on the registry divided by their member-months. It is typically ten to twenty times higher than average medical costs.

Overall hospital admissions per one thousand is another basic outcome measure of the economic efficiency of an MCO. Because hospitalizations are the largest single category of medical expenses, the more good quality care that can be provided with modest use of hospitals, the more successful the risk-bearing organization will be. This metric is calculated by taking the actual number of hospital admissions for a given month and expressing it on an annualized basis for one thousand members. Organizations usually report different figures for those insured under "commercial" managed care plans, and those over sixty-five under managed Medicare risk plans.

The *Status One hospital admission rate* measures the proportion of patients on this registry hospitalized each month. Because Status One care is fundamentally an admissions-avoidance strategy, admissions are expected to trend downward over time. Prior to redesigning care for these frail and clinically ill members, admission rates in MCOs will be in the 15 to 20 percent range per month. After proactive care management is introduced, rates as low as 5 percent have been observed, and that rate is the benchmark. The difference between current performance and the benchmark represents millions of dollars in medical expenditures to even a midsized group practice at financial risk.

A closely related metric is *hospital days per thousand members*. Dividing days per thousand members by admissions per thousand members yields the average length of stay. Much effort has been expended on shortening hospital stays. The chief impact of Status One care planning is avoiding hospitalization, as reflected in overall hospital admissions per thousand members.

The *Status One hospital utilization rate* is the portion of monthly hospitalizations attributed to Status One members. It most often begins in the 25 to 40 percent range for all admissions. It confirms that a population-based health management program is concentrating its efforts on the smallest feasible group contributing disproportionately to high-cost care.

It is fair to say that no MCO has yet seen the full extent of economic and clinical achievements possible because no system of care has fully reached the limits of innovation and interventions on behalf of its Status One members.

Process Measures

Status One population prevalence is the portion of a managed care membership meeting Status One criteria during any month. In mixed senior and commercial populations, this consistently runs in the range of 0.5 to 1.0 percent. The larger figure occurs when relatively more seniors are managed care members. Status One population prevalence among seniors can be 1.5 to 2 percent.

Members will join the highest-risk group as an equivalent number leave. Although overall numbers tend to be stable, individual groups and practices often differ in the proportion of Status One patients they serve. It is important to derive population prevalence in order to arrive at the right number of care managers and to assign them to places where the highest-risk patients are being served.

The *care plan completion rate* represents the percentage of current Status One patients who have completed assessments and operational care plans. It is a constant challenge to establish and keep care plans up to date with a dynamic population. This important process measure is a useful indicator of the effectiveness of the care planning effort.

Acuity levels, as discussed earlier, represent the professional judgment of care managers and PCPs on the likelihood of and time frame for hospitalization of patients already identified as high risk by the computerized modeling. As explained in Chapter Five, acuities run from 1, hospitalization likely within three months, to 5, hospitalization possible two or more years in the future. Acuity levels provide a way to triage patients and to determine the intensity of their care plans even within the Status One registry. Taken as a cross-sectional prevalence value, acuity level becomes an important process measure and means of ensuring that the highest acuity Status One patients are fully attended.

Functional status as a cross-sectional metric is the average prevalence of measured values across all the care plans in effect at a given time. The most useful single functional status measure is the global well-being question from SF-36s and similar instruments: "Considering everything, how would you rate your health?" The scale runs from 1, poor, up to 5, excellent. The care manager records the numeric result at the time of initial assessment. The question is repeated each time the health action plan is updated. Functional status is the single most effective way of assuring that Status One interventions are not achieving economic efficiencies at the cost of decreased well-being. On the level of the individual patient, it has less meaning, with the exception of a "poor" response, which is a risk factor in itself of potential clinical instability.

Potential Measures

A large number of alternate measures for managing interventions for subpopulations exist. The advantage to the measures already discussed here is their usefulness to real-world administrative and clinical leaders, their simplicity, and the fact that they are familiar as a precise subset of current cost and utilization statistics for the overall population. Following a pragmatic approach to all aspects of population-based care management is prudent in an era of scarce resources.

Other possible measures can be envisioned. Many are of a research nature, associated with redirecting medical management across diseases and toward the patients with a near-term likelihood of high resource use.

We caution MCO leaders to include research metrics only to the extent that they have dedicated grants and budgets for researching issues arising from programs accepted into their organizations. Although research metrics address valid questions and areas of collateral interest, we have judged them not the best choices given considerations of cost, timeliness, or relevance to leading a major clinical improvement initiative. Compared with the seven Status One financial, utilization, and process measures, the alternate measures are not essential for achieving results with an economy of effort.

Among the additional measures is a *cohort analysis*, which tracks the experience of fixed groups of patients over time. Although of considerable research interest, the experience of these groups has little management or operational impact. Rather, focus should remain on the efficiency of care provided to, and the functional status of, *current* Status One members. The cross-sectional prevalence metrics described above are recommended Status One measures. Standard MCO utilization statistics are all cross-sectional prevalence metrics.

Member satisfaction, another possible metric, is not recommended as a routine measure for subpopulations of patients. The meaning of such numbers is suspect. Patients whose care is often fragmented are bound to be more satisfied when dedicated nurses or social workers customize care collaboratively with them. Baseline values will not be available. Results will not change a Status

One intervention. Status One patients are so few that whatever their satisfaction levels are or become, the impact will be lost among the larger membership. In time, as health care delivery systems redesign the process of care to respond to the needs of Status One patients, feedback on patient satisfaction will help to identify continuous improvements.

Measures based on the individual care manager or provider are possible. Included are *functional status by individual care manager* and *hospitalization and other rates by individual provider*. When so few individuals are cared for by any one professional and when their clinical situations are so varied, individual statistics of this sort will have little meaning. In like fashion, *single disease incidence* among Status One members, *functional status beyond the aggregate measure, patient-level clinical outcomes*, and *mortality* will have little impact on managing and leading a Status One program.

· · · · · · ·

In this chapter a set of measures were identified for managing and monitoring a Status One population. Comparable statistics are useful for each of the common disease registries; doing so puts diverse clinical interventions on a common platform for monitoring initiatives and demonstrating results.

Part III

. . . .

Alternate Approaches to
Medical Management

9

Theory of the Case
Varied Ways to Identify High-Risk People

This chapter surveys the methods available to leaders of MCOs for stratifying members according to risk and medical needs. Chapter Three described a model for predicting future high costs, a method culminating in registries of Status One members.

Experience and Published Papers

The published literature on predicting high-risk patients in general populations is limited (Corrigan and Martin, 1992). Studies address particular diagnoses (Berkman, Miller, Holmes, and Boander, 1991; Crane and others, 1992), seniors (Burns and Nichols, 1991), or results of functional status instruments. There is no agreement on how far back one must go to collect input data, which data are important, or whether administrative information is necessary or sufficient.

Published studies that address stratification on the basis of future clinical and economic risk include populations that are often preselected. Literature is more plentiful for the elderly (Fehtke, Smith, and Johnson, 1986) than for children (Anderson and Steinberg, 1995). HMO insurer data follow their product lines—Medicare senior risk products, commercial offerings, and Medicaid managed care plans.

Capitated health care delivery systems, including staff, group, and IPA models, most often serve patients from multiple insurers and include multiple products for each insurer. Published results on population-segmentation methodologies in such organizations have not been available, although the challenge to these systems is to manage a membership of many different ages and with many different insurance plans. Predictive modeling for clinical complexity and associated high costs can be most challenging in these environments. The incentives to reorient the medical management strategies toward high-risk population health management are just as great in a capitated delivery system as in a health plan.

Identification Methods

Population segmentation is a requisite building block for high-risk population health management. Methods for identifying high-risk members include provider designations, demographics, questionnaires, prior utilization, pharmacy data, specific diagnoses, high cost, and patterns of care.

Provider Designations

In Chapter Two we first encountered patients who are viewed by their health care providers as high users of costly services. They are sometimes called members of the "frequent flier club," after their frequent utilization of hospital wards, intensive care units, and emergency rooms. The field of the observers' vision limits such a designation. Providers are familiar with those patients whom they see often or about whom they are concerned, but they do not know the Status One patients with whom they are not familiar. To the ambulatory-care nurse, the "frequent fliers" are patients frequently appearing on the physician's office schedule. To the discharge planner, high users are often found in the hospital. To the ER physician, such high users are patients who frequently need emergency care. On the basis of future demand for high-intensity services, many of these people may be Status One, but without a systematic process for assessing their current care and patterns of care, health care professionals have difficulty objectively focusing their efforts.

Typically, designation of Status One type patients by clinicians overlooks half of those at high risk. Those missed encompass a variety of people who skip their appointments, members unknown to their PCPs, patients whose care is provided by multiple specialists without an integrated care plan, and users of episodic care. Only a systematic and consistent method of identifying Status One and other at-risk patients can produce measurable results and be systematically improved. Anecdotal identification is not a process that can be characterized or measured, and it is amenable to neither analysis nor improvement.

Otherwise precise and compassionate clinicians frequently refer to "train wrecks," "accidents waiting to happen," "patients waiting to crash land in the ER," and use similar colorful analogies when describing high-risk patients. Powerlessness and therapeutic nihilism underlie such labels. The current approach to health care offers only a few alternatives for Status One patients—inpatient care, ER care, or brief office visits, for which the inherent complexity of their situation makes them poorly suited. It is no wonder that even compassionate health care professionals see the highest-risk patients as needing more than they can possibly do for them. Yet, as these needs continue to be unmet, the system and the patient pay dearly.

Demographics

Another method for identifying high-risk members is to select demographic characteristics such as age. Income is a demographic item usually not directly available to the managed care executive, but it can be inferred in the case of Medicaid members. Age and sex are always found in membership data. Examples of the use of demographic selection criteria include offering a comprehensive geriatric assessment to all members older than eighty, targeting a high-risk pregnancy program to Medicaid managed care members, or providing an osteoporosis-prevention program for all women over forty. The Health Care Financing Agency (HCFA) employs demographics by setting its county-specific capitation rates for managed medical care higher for seniors aged eighty or above. In each case, one or two demographic characteristics are used to define a group of people in order to combat a health condition common to them. Based only on age and birthrates, Medicaid members and families are logical beneficiaries of prenatal-care programs. In the case of HCFA, demographic characteristics provide a rate-setting mechanism that attempts to fairly capitate HMOs for higher anticipated costs.

Although demographics are the most accessible and obvious way to stratify a population, they are unsatisfactory for identifying the group of patients at highest risk; the numbers are impracticably high. Age alone is not a particularly useful predictor of high risk. More promising are demographics employed in combination with other clinical information available within the HMO or health care delivery system.

Questionnaires

Questionnaires have contributed both to stratifying managed care populations and to assessing outcomes across diagnoses. Questionnaires typically are completed by patients and reflect their view of their own health. The consumer view had been historically lacking from decades of fee-for-service medicine. The Rand Corporation's pioneering Medical Outcomes Studies made great strides during the 1980s in rectifying the absence of standardized, quantified, and reproducible measures of consumer health and outcomes (Stewart and others, 1989). The wellness and health-promotion movement also fostered the development of health risk appraisals, with early applications directed to self-insured employee groups.

The questionnaires with the most extensive validation literature are the Short Form 36 and the Short Form 12 (Ware, Snow,

Kosinski, and Gandek, 1995). The P_{ra} (Boult and others, 1993; Boult, Pacala, and Boult, 1995; Pacala, Boult, and Boult, 1995; Pacala, Boult, Reed, and Aliberti, 1997) is also notable for attempting to predict near-term, repeat hospitalization.

The advantage of a questionnaire is that it provides a view of health and well-being that comes directly from the patient and also provides information that is otherwise unavailable in the medical records. Questionnaires often include, for example, screening questions for depression, activities of daily living, and nutritional status. For new members of an MCO or medical practice, questionnaire information is the only kind that may be available.

Several considerations make patient screening questionnaires less desirable for identifying high-risk patients. Effort must be expended printing and distributing questionnaires. The response rate is always a concern. Subgroups of greatest concern—people with disabilities in long-term care facilities for example—have a low response rate. It takes time to compile the incoming data and to translate them into clinically useful form. Because Status One patients in particular form an unstable group, questionnaires would have to be administered frequently in order to be current for the highest-risk patients. Given the various limitations of questionnaire use in a large population, it is worth noting that equivalent accuracy can be obtained from far more accessible administrative databases (Coleman and others, 1998).

Utilization Rates

Utilization data include claims for inpatient care and for ambulatory and emergency services. Claims paid are financial records of clinical services for which health plans have paid on behalf of their members. Provider organizations generate charges for services for which they bill health care payers. Although their primary purpose is for financial administration, considerable effort has been made to code clinical diagnoses (*International Classification of Diseases*, 1998), procedures (Kirchner and others, 1996), and pharmaceuticals

(Cardinale, 1998). Adapting this data, already encoded in electronic form, is an attractive approach (Ellis and Ash, 1995/1996).

Issues can be raised about utilization data. Insurers typically have a lag between when they receive a claim for services and when they pay it. Delays in claims payment can often be three months. Provider charges are more timely but less accurate. Many charges will be modified or denied, and services outside the network are not included. Authorization data are the most timely but are even less complete and accurate. For example, tentative diagnoses made at hospital admission turn out to be erroneous once tests and the further clinical course become known.

For provider groups serving multiple payers, the most common and most rapidly increasing HMO arrangement with providers nationally, a practical means of integrating their experience across payers is necessary for population-based management of their members, for whom they bear financial risk. Most organizations have not yet exploited potential clinical uses of their utilization data.

Pharmacy Data

Pharmacy claims data typically include the name of the drug, dosage, dispensed amount, and payments. Like medical utilization data, claims are generated for administrative and financial reasons, but contain important clinical information. For example, diabetics can be identified by codes from the International Classification of Diseases, 9th Edition (ICD9), appearing on their inpatient and outpatient claims. In a capitated delivery system, where record keeping on ambulatory patients can be lax, pharmaceutical claims for insulin and oral hypoglycemic drugs may be the best means for establishing a registry of diabetic patients. Even patients who have not been seen by their clinician in many months and are lost to clinical follow-up will be renewing their prescriptions for insulin. Pharmacy data have the additional benefit of implying risk stratification within a disease. Diabetics on insulin are, in general, more seriously afflicted than those on oral agents.

Pharmacy data can be adapted for identifying high-risk patients (Bishop and Macarounas-Kirchman, 1997). Papers in the scientific literature focus on screening members for poly-pharmacy (the simultaneous administration of multiple drugs in different therapeutic classes) as a risk factor for future complex care. Use of specific drugs and combinations of agents can serve as a proxy for knowing the clinical diagnoses (Clark and others, 1995). Surveillance for renewals of important chronic-disease medications is another creative use of pharmacy data. In some situations, pharmacy claims data may be the most available of the electronic databases. In the case of pharmaceutical benefit managers (PBMs), intermediaries between payers and retail pharmacies for numerous HMOs and self-insured companies, pharmacy claims may be the only electronically encoded data at their disposal.

Several issues temper the exclusive use of pharmacy claims data to predict at-risk populations. Retail pharmacies file claims to get paid rather than for more precise, clinical uses. For example, often the subscriber number, which is required for reimbursement, is recorded accurately, while member number, which is needed for clinical purposes, is missing or incorrect. Other practical situations can limit the availability and use of pharmacy data. PBMs vary widely in their ability and willingness to provide clinical initiatives for HMOs and provider groups based on the data they have accumulated.

Specific Diagnoses

Diagnoses can be determined directly from claims or inferred from other sources, for example dialysis treatments and vascular shunt placement for end-stage renal disease (Burns, Seddon, Saul, and Zeidel, 1998). Managed care initiatives based on disease are the norm for high-risk patients. Disease management initiatives are the subject of Chapter Eleven; the challenges of comorbidities and psychosocial issues blunt the effectiveness of single-disease programs. Additionally, no one diagnosis or combination of diagnoses dominates among Status One patients.

High Cost

A history of high cost is often taken as a criterion for considering patients at risk for future complications (Kongstvedt, 1993). Inclusion in catastrophic case management at HMOs is frequently triggered once $100,000 or $50,000 has been spent.

The problem with accepting past high cost as a predictor of high-risk patients is the extent, usually untested, to which past cost experience is a predictor of the future. The natural history of the condition being treated may be advanced. The ability to intervene meaningfully may be limited. In some organizations stop-loss insurance engages at a predetermined level, diffusing the incentives to manage the costs of catastrophic cases.

Patterns of Care

Predictive algorithms for Status One patient registries (Forman, Kelliher, and Wood, 1997) were described in Chapter Three. This multifactorial, continuous-flow approach depends on patterns of care derived from membership, claims, pharmacy data, and, if available, laboratory data.

Comparison of Predictive Models

Direct comparisons of predictive models are difficult, although stratifying according to risk is a requirement of high-risk population health management. Table 9.1 provides an objective comparison of some of the high-risk identification methods. This table is based on research at a large multipayer IDS with one hundred thousand managed care members. The IDS is at full financial risk for these members, of whom approximately 89 percent have commercial insurance, 5 percent are covered by Medicare, and 6 percent are in Medicaid managed care plans.

Two years of historical data were used in the comparison. A typical variant of each identification model was applied to data for the

Table 9.1. Alternative Predictive Models Applied to an Integrated Delivery System's Managed Care Population.

Predictive Method	Criteria Applied to Base Year	# Identified as High Risk per 1,000	$PMPY in Following Year
Questionnaire	P_{ra} top quartile	250	2,560
Utilization			
Prior hospitalization	2+ admissions	41.9	4,145
Outpatient visits	10+ visits	198.8	2,476
ER visits	3+ visits	9.7	4,587
Drug-Use Patterns			
Poly-pharmacy	6+ different prescriptions	118	2,893
Clinical Diagnoses			
Congestive heart failure	Diagnosis	5.7	8,743
Chronic obstructive pulmonary disease	Diagnosis	41.4	2,096
Adult respiratory failure	Diagnosis	2.3	3,662
Newborn respiratory failure	Diagnosis	0.9	1,599
Oncology	Diagnosis	45.2	3,177
Oncology w/chemotherapy	Diagnosis	5.0	7,198
Renal insufficiency	Diagnosis	3.5	6,177
Catastrophic Cases (prior stop-loss)	$50,000 cost	1.4	18,557
Status One	Patterns of care	5.8	27,480

Note: Figures are for a fully capitated IDS. $N = 100,000$.

first year to yield the number of people identified as high risk. The actual dollars expended per person during the subsequent year ($PMPY) were calculated from claims for all services divided by member-months. $PMPY can be viewed as a basic financial measure of the ability to discern clinically complicated and costly cases before they occur. The objective was to determine a subpopulation of manageable size (high-risk patients per one thousand members) where the future cost ($PMPY) was great enough to justify aggressive care management and where the opportunity to affect these costs was significant.

Administering a typical questionnaire (Boult, 1995) would identify a top quartile of patients costing four times more than the bottom quartile. Applied to this population, 250 of every 1,000 members would be placed in the highest risk category. These people each expended $2,560 per year compared with the $1,750 average across the entire population. Twenty-five thousand people identified in this way would be far too many for incremental care management.

Prior hospitalizations were a more effective predictor of high risk. Taking two or more hospitalizations in the previous year, a criterion widely used by case managers, 41.9 patients per 1,000 would be identified as high risk, and costs were $4,145 PMPY in the following year. In a population of 100,000 managed care members, over 4,000 would be identified as high risk, a figure still too high to enable proactive intervention.

Frequent outpatient visits also proves to be a poor criterion for identifying high-risk patients. If providers are asked to identify their highest-risk patients, they name a disproportionate number of the worried well, high outpatient users whom they see often but who do not have a huge impact on overall medical costs because they seldom require intensive hospitalization. This method would identify 198.8 patients for every 1,000 members. Average costs were $2,476 during the subsequent year, indicating predictive capability only a little better than that of a questionnaire-based strategy.

Using poly-pharmacy and specific diagnoses as the criteria yields only modest improvements in predicting the at-risk population at a manageable size or in predicting medical costs incurred in the outcome year. Among chronic diseases, only CHF identifies relatively few patients at high average future costs. Catastrophic cases set at $50,000 in the base year seems promising, tempered by the observation that subsequent costs are lower at $18,557 PMPY. The majority of costs have been expended prior to identification, but the potential ongoing effects on this very small group are sizable.

The Status One approach, which identifies patients using patterns of care, produces 5.8 patients per 1,000 members and an average of $27,480 PMPY. The patient numbers are small enough to pursue intensive care management, while unmanaged costs are large enough to warrant constructive interventions to preempt the need for high-acuity, expensive care.

· · · · · · · ·

This chapter surveyed means of stratifying a population for future clinical frailty and associated high costs. Approaches include provider judgment, questionnaire, prior utilization of services, pharmacy use, specific diagnoses, and prior high cost. Status One, a multifactorial approach, yields an attractive combination of relatively small numbers of people likely to incur very high PMPM costs in the coming year.

10

Intervening on Behalf of the
Severely Afflicted

Case Management

High-risk population health management obtains results by working with one patient at a time. The key human resource for engaging high-risk patients is care managers. Case management is an existing function in most MCOs (Quick, 1997). It is important for leaders and practitioners to distinguish case management from care management as they contemplate gaps in their organizational capabilities and how best to address them.

Until this point, the rationale for segmenting a population, the characterization of a small group of costly and challenging patients, the care management process (which incorporates psychosocial issues) for Status One patients, and program metrics have been explained. As described in Chapters Five, Six, and Seven, care management for Status One patients supplements the usual medical care. Through assessing the situations of clients at highest future risk of developing clinical complexities and working collaboratively with these clients, care managers are able to develop and execute customized health action plans. The aim is to raise functional status and thereby reduce, on a population basis, the need for the highest acuity care.

Distinguishing Case Management from Care Management

The nursing profession does not yet have a uniform nomenclature for case management. What we describe here as care management is an extension of third-generation case management (Thorn, 1993), including managing the needs of a small panel of patients across the continuum on the basis of predictive modeling, systematic approaches to psychosocial issues, and the measurement of population-based outcomes. Rather than getting lost in nomenclature, we find it useful to distinguish current case management practice from the essential attributes needed for the care of Status One patients (see Table 10.1).

Clients and Patients

One piece of nomenclature is often insisted on by nurses and social workers—calling the people they serve *clients*. Status One people can be clients when on a care manager's panel. They certainly are *patients* too, in that they present the most complicated and unstable clinical situations of anyone cared for by physicians. They are

Table 10.1. Comparison of Case Management and Care Management.

Case Management	Care Management
Inclusion by dollar threshold and large size of case	Inclusion by prediction of risk
Care coupled to setting	Continuum of care
Episodic	Longitudinal
Patient as object	Patient as collaborator
Patient refusal ends process	Patient refusal does not end coordination of medical care
Estimated savings	Real population savings
Clinical outcomes uncertain	Population acuity and functional status measured

also *members* of managed care plans. The term *client* enlivens nurses and social workers but can puzzle physicians. Labeling a person a *patient* can place some listeners into a physician's mind-set. Labeling that person a *member* means something else to administrators and unites nurses, social workers, and physicians in defiance.

Above all, the goal is to recognize and manage high-risk people well. Distinguishing case from care management is useful only to the extent that it enables thought and actions devoted to improving care for Status One patients.

Inclusion Criteria

Case management begins with patient referrals. Case management typically is applied to people who have incurred high costs over the past year (often $25,000 to $50,000), who have catastrophic conditions like AIDS or multiple organ transplants, or who have diagnoses of particular interest, such as CHF. Often the field of eligible members is large and the process of case selection haphazard.

By contrast, care management for high-risk patients begins with a registry of members who are predicted to incur high costs during the following year. *Population-based* means that all such members are included. Costs are an outcome rather than an inclusion criterion.

Setting

Case management, as it is currently practiced, is coupled to setting, meaning the physical facility (physician's office, hospital, nursing home). Clinical horizons extend only as far as the borders of the sponsoring facility and perhaps a bit beyond. Inevitably, purview is limited by the interests of the employing organization. Table 10.2 captures the limited scope of case managers whose practice is shaped by institutional strategies and requirements.

Care management requires both influencing care delivered across all settings and affecting social issues contributing to high risk. Such "care across the continuum" is a staple of case management, but it is rarely encountered in practice. For care of Status One

Table 10.2. Case Management Settings and Scope of Activities.

Setting	General Scope of Work
Inpatient general ward	Discharge planning and concurrent review
Inpatient specialty services	Discharge planning and concurrent review related to the cause of hospitalization
Home care	Case management while on the home-care service
Obstetrics	Case management for duration of high-risk pregnancy
Outpatient	High users of outpatient services
Insurers	Utilization management and utilization review within covered benefits
Disease management programs	Care for patients with a particular diagnosis
PBMs	Use of preferred drugs
Employer-based care	Return-to-work and catastrophic case management for self-insured companies

patients to be fully integrated and effective, it must provide services, or work closely with those who do, in every setting patients may find themselves part of. MCOs, at financial risk for all patient care, have both the means and the incentive to work across the continuum.

Time Frame

For care to be extended from one setting to another, the time frame must be longitudinal. Having case managers work toward limiting inpatient stays is a ubiquitous element of MCOs and hospitals concerned about managing within Disease Related Group targets. The activities of case managers in these settings have short time frames and are limited to hospital discharge planning. Some case managers close their cases as the patient passes beyond the hospital door. Other managers might be involved for up to thirty days to prevent "bounce-backs," unplanned rehospitalizations.

Patient Focus

Case managers must perform their work quickly, for they only have available the time the patient is served by their institution. Such "drive-by" encounters cannot possibly enable case managers to delve into the clinical complexities and social situations of Status One patients. The patient is more an object to be moved on from an episode of care than a person who can collaborate with health professionals to improve his or her functional status over time.

Care management for Status One patients is designed to engage patients' own goals and priorities in order to improve their health status from their starting condition. Even modest gains, when linked to what is truly important to an individual, can have gratifying results in reversing the trend toward the highest acuity and most expensive care.

Patient Refusals

The universe of possible case manager–patient relationships is extremely large. At one extreme, the patient may refuse to work with the case manager. At that point, the traditional case management relationship stops.

Status One patient refusals are handled quite differently. Although the full benefit accruing from addressing the Status One aims as prioritized by the patient cannot be realized without active collaboration, medical care, at least, can continue to be coordinated. Coordination of medical care is the one aim that is the most direct responsibility of the health delivery system and is the financial imperative of risk-retaining MCOs.

In addition, because care is longitudinal, the member can be approached later to solicit active participation in the care planning process. Many will reverse their initial refusals and may ultimately be pleased by the organization's continued interest and the care manager's gentle persistence.

Savings Calculations

Case managers spend a portion of time estimating the cost benefits of their interventions. Doing so involves costing out a plan of care that the care manager has specified. Next comes a subjective process of estimating what the care would have cost if case management were not performed. The difference is presented as the cost savings generated by case management (Schore, Brown, Cheh, and Schneider, 1997).

Such calculations can be viewed as cost-avoidance estimates. "Soft money" of this sort is difficult for leaders to reconcile to actual organizational expenditures and financial performance. Allied issues also conspire to weaken the impact of such analyses. An unproductive dynamic ensues. Case managers put increasing effort into producing cost-avoidance estimates that managers inherently mistrust. The more effort put into costing pursuits, the less time devoted to engaging patients in care plans.

High-risk population health management bypasses the issue by relieving care managers of cost estimation while monitoring the actual performance of this subpopulation in a way that provides for increased accuracy in managing the practice or enterprise. Once patients are identified in the high-risk patient registry, data on actual performance, including cost, are derived from services rendered to them while they are Status One. High-risk population health management obviates the need for estimates and is an exact subset of the monthly financial and utilization figures that all MCOs use to manage their business. Chapter 9 expounded on the rationale for and derivation of Status One population-based outcome statistics.

Certainty of Outcomes

Case management can report only estimated cost and hospital utilization for their clients because its population base is ill-defined. For example, asthmatics requiring maintenance steroids have aggregated clinical measures and utilization statistics produced with special effort by a disease management program, but it is difficult to correlate these data with the overall impact on the cost of care for all asthmatics in the population. By incorporating functional status tools into the assessment process, Status One methods can readily extract population cross-sectional pictures of functional status. Full questionnaires are available to perform targeted evaluations of further subsets that might be involved in an incremental disease initiative.

Once a care management group is defined on a population basis, the same kind of economic and clinical measurements that are applied to managed care memberships in general can now be applied to high-risk members or any diseased-based subpopulation. The outcomes are as accurate and as certain as the populationwide measures that leaders commonly use to manage the enterprise. Such metrics compare favorably to estimates of fragmented case management groupings or measured outcomes for small subsets of the population, whose relationship to the overall membership and "bottom line" is unknown.

Staffing

Staffing of case management is an issue of practical concern for leaders. Unfortunately, the content and approach to case management have been standardized to only a limited extent, and analyses of benchmark practices and staffing ratios are largely subjective. In many organizations, case managers attempting longitudinal care for high-risk patients will have no direct patient contact and little time for understanding the patients' real needs. Low-intensity case management, like telephone calls by PBMs reminding patients about medication, may work well at staffing ratios of one to several hundred. At the other extreme, case loads of twenty to forty permit time for home visits and close personal interest. Such staffing is characteristic of disease management for advanced states of AIDS and New York Heart Association Class IV cardiac patients. Staffing levels adequate for the close monitoring and management of the

Status One patient result in case loads of forty to sixty. From a planning perspective, it is best to settle on the approach and professional content of care management (Chapters Five, Six, and Seven) that best fit the organization's needs and only then to address staffing levels as an implementation issue (Chapter Four).

Requisite Skills

There is little consensus on the combination of education and skills needed to be an effective case manager. Six organizations (Table 10.3) currently offer certifications in case management, each requiring specific combinations of formal education, experience, and ability.

In contrast to the skills needed by case managers, care management relies heavily on managers who have empathic people skills for relating to patients, creativity for developing care plans, and diplomacy in dealing with clinicians and other providers in the health care system. An ability to learn about and actively incorporate psychosocial issues into care plans is also necessary.

The current experience in both delivery systems and insurance settings indicates the necessity of emphasizing care manager competencies over formal credentials. Extensive prior job experience with episodic forms of case management can lessen rapid adaptation to and high performance in serving Status One patient panels. Too much of an orientation to rules and limits, as can occur from operating strictly within a benefit structure, can constrain creative solutions in Status One care plans.

Either nurses or social workers can be care managers; the competencies for the role, as outlined here, should be paramount in hiring decisions:

- The ideal care manager is able to:

    Communicate concisely and clearly both orally and
    in writing

Table 10.3. Case Manager Certifications.

Credentialing Body and Name of Certification	Eligibility	Contact Information
Healthcare Quality Certification Board of the National Association for Healthcare Quality Certified Professional in Healthcare Quality (CPHQ)	Minimum: associate's degree Includes nursing and medical records	P.O. Box 1880 San Gabriel, CA 91778 818-286-8074 www.nahq.org/cphq.htm
National Academy of Certified Care Managers Care Manager Certification (CMC)	Master's degree in nursing, social work, psychology, or related field	3389 Sheridan Street Suite 170 Hollywood, FL 33021
Rehabilitation Nursing Certification Board Certified Rehabilitation Registered Nurse (CRRN)	Registered Nurse	4700 West Lake Avenue Glenview, IL 60025 800-229-7530
Commission for Case Manager Certification Certified Case Manager (CCM)	Postsecondary education in a related field	1835 Rohling Road Suite E Rolling Meadows, IL 60008 847-818-0292
Certification of Disability Management Specialists Certified Disability Management Specialist (CDMS)	Registered Nurse, master's, or doctoral degree	1835 Rohling Road Suite E Rolling Meadows, IL 60008 847-394-2106
National Board of Certification in Continuity of Care Advanced Continuity of Care Certification (A-CCC)	Bachelor's degree	7313 Southview Court Fairfax Station, VA 22039 860-586-7525

Perform multiple activities simultaneously

Manage details

Hold providers and ancillaries accountable for care plan activities

Operate with little direct supervision

Conceptualize his or her role as being within a system and seek ways to improve it

Be assertive in clarifying points and actions with clinicians

- The ideal care manager demonstrates:

  Ease in working with physicians

  Creativity in formulating care plans from assessment and clinical information

  Comfort with, or willingness to learn, new technology

  Knowledge concerning relevant resources within the organization and in the community

  Openness to innovative approaches

  Willingness to participate in ongoing learning

- The ideal care manager is:

  Respected within the organization for his or her opinions and recommendations

  Patient-centered rather than strictly oriented toward rules and limits

- The ideal care manager has the following credentials:

  Bachelor of Science in Nursing (B.S.N.) or Master of Social Work (M.S.W.)

  Current professional license

Additional credentials and experience if working with particular sorts of patients—for example, cardiac rehabilitation, geriatric care, or renal dialysis

Prior experience with direct patient contact and the provision of care

If social workers manage Status One patients, they have to have nurses readily available to advise on some of the clinical aspects of care planning. With the more traditional model of nurse case managers, social work advice is frequently needed and must be available to and used by the nurse care managers.

Opportunities for Professional Contributions

High-risk population health management challenges professionals to realize the long-standing promise of patient-centered care across the continuum. Thoughtfully carried out, health management is essential in MCOs retaining financial risk. Professionals who adopt new approaches and discard unproductive case management practices will be revered by clients and valued by clinicians and leaders, whose success with managed care will depend on them.

· · · · · · ·

In this chapter case management, as currently practiced, has been contrasted with the practice and skills required of professionals managing Status One clients.

. . . .

11

Intervening by Clinical Condition
Disease Management

Because disease management is the major alternative clinical approach to high-risk population health management, leaders, clinicians, and care managers must understand its rationale, strengths, and limitations. Disease management and high-risk population management are not mutually exclusive; rather, they arise from different and complementary strategies.

Disease management has an important role. Indeed, many MCOs have successfully implemented disease-oriented programs. The challenges are to integrate disease management programs in support of population health management, to monitor the economic benefits, to expand those programs that prove successful, and to scale back those that do not.

Definition

Disease management is an umbrella term for a variety of clinical programs that seek to standardize and improve the care process for members afflicted with particular diseases and conditions (Ellrodt and others, 1997). Initiatives typically utilize tools from the quality movement, most often clinical guidelines and measured outcomes (Epstein and Sherwood, 1996). These programs are a phenomenon of managed care.

These are the common attributes of disease management programs:

- They address conditions of concern to payers.

  High costs

  Large membership involvement

  Opportunity for economic efficiencies

- They limit undesirable practice variations.

- They are used for cases where clinical guidelines exist or can be developed.

- They orchestrate a variety of interventions.

  Least intense: general membership education

  Most intense: clinical contact and aggressive case management

- They measure outcomes.

Typically disease management programs address issues that are important to payers either directly as expressed in NCQA's HEDIS measures or indirectly through the promise of economic efficiencies (Harris, 1996). A particular diagnosis that exhibits high costs with an opportunity for savings and that involves large numbers of members is an attractive candidate for disease management.

Undesirable or costly practice variations also point to diseases that might benefit from a standardized program. These can range from high Cesarean rates to low prescriptions for angiotensin converting enzyme inhibitors for people afflicted with CHF.

Interventions of disease management programs can be truly diverse. The familiar patient-education leaflets can be cast as disease management, as can the provision of direct and specialized case management services for heart-failure patients and carved-out networks of subcapitated specialty-care providers (Blumenthal and Buntin, 1998).

Finally, most disease management programs offer some outcomes measures encompassing a combination of clinical markers, economics, and patient satisfaction.

Drivers

Disease management as a movement has been fueled by diverse factors, including HEDIS clinical quality measures, pharmaceutical companies, investors, and unexplained therapy variations.

Use of Disease Management as a Clinical Paradigm

Disease management has grown in popularity in tandem with the growth of managed care membership. As cost competition continues, clinical leaders have been challenged to cut costs and simultaneously maintain or improve quality. Trained in a clinical paradigm, they find it natural to single out diseases one by one for improvement efforts. HEDIS clinical measures fuel the movement as they expand from the simple presence or absence of preventive measures to the diagnosis, follow-up, and control of common conditions.

Marketing Strategies of Drug Companies

Pharmaceutical manufacturers and PBMs have propelled much of the disease management movement. Traditionally they introduced new drugs to a fee-for-service (FFS) clinical community eager for novelty and insulated from cost considerations. With the shift to managed care, the challenge has become to constructively engage leaders who control managed care formularies and to convince them not only of superior clinical efficacy but of the overall cost advantage.

Encouragement of the Financial Community

The financial community has a keen interest in disease management companies. Like the pharmaceutical industry, venture capital has fueled the growth of this sector. Meanwhile MCO leaders have developed a jaundiced attitude to claims of cost savings coming from disease management initiatives.

Requirements of Self-Insured Payers

On occasion a special interest of a large commercial payer will spawn disease management initiatives. Johnson & Johnson and Du Pont's wellness initiatives began as internal programs for employees and have subsequently been offered to other payers. Some payers will prompt HMOs serving their employees to supply a particular disease management program selected on the basis of its importance to a particular working population. Examples encompass not only the major chronic illnesses afflicting the general population but specialized issues such as teenage drug abuse in dependents and diseases of personal interest to the organization's leaders. Delivery systems can face challenges in executing such programs for a number of companies simultaneously because the members of each of the companies constitute only a modest part of a delivery system's members.

Use of Clinical Guidelines

Disease management programs borrow heavily from assembly-line production theory (see Table 11.1). The analogy is not close in every area. Long implementation times and the complexities of suc-

Table 11.1. Production Analogy.

Assembly Line	Disease Management
Production line	Guidelines and DRGs
Unskilled workers	Staff vary by disease
Aims to increase uniformity and decrease variation	Aims to decrease variation through use of guidelines
Short implementation time	Long implementation time
Measurable outcomes	Measurable outcomes

cessfully instituting workflows and clinical guidelines distinguish medical care from the industrial experience.

Disease management programs, like assembly lines, are attempts to limit unnecessary, unexplained, and costly variation. Disease management accomplishes this aim through the use of standard approaches and clinical guidelines (Field and Lohr, 1992). A veritable guideline industry has arisen in response (Vibbert, Migdail, Strickland, and Youngs, 1994; American Medical Association, 1998).

Guidelines, pathways, best practices, and similar standards date from early advocacy of clinical quality. Hospital services have been characterized as a progression from inputs to outputs, posing challenges of implementing the best, most efficient practices (Codman, 1914; Codman, 1916; Donabedian, 1966) and adherence to guidelines. Diagnosis Related Groups, best known now as an inpatient reimbursement device, were created to group like inpatient services together in order to optimize care according to product lines (Fetter, 1991). Such approaches resonate strongly with the mapping of customers and supplier chains and the workflow diagrams encouraged by the industrial quality movement (Deming, 1986).

Guidelines have taken on a life of their own. Clinicians can be coaxed into discussing optimal practices and will do so at great length. The results of such deliberations are variable (Weingarten and Ellrodt, 1992). Some guidelines are based on randomized, double-blind clinical research and strong clinical outcomes. Most are based on the consensus opinions of whoever was sitting down at the discussion. At another extreme are guidelines admonishing frequent referrals to subspecialty care; they reinforce FFS practice patterns without evidence of efficacy.

Guidelines can be challenging to implement (Berman, 1992). Many of the clinical end points are not electronically accessible, a situation resulting in cumbersome data acquisition and long periods between interventions and the assessment of outcomes. Clinical interventions, such as pharmacotherapy of moderate hypertension as a way of lowering the risk for strokes and myocardial infarction, can have long latencies.

The challenge posed by guidelines is that they are designed for the usual or average case. They default to the clinician's judgment in complicated and comorbid situations. Unfortunately, just such situations characterize Status One patients.

Comparison with Care Management

Care of the sort that follows from high-risk population health management diverges in a number of areas from disease management (see Table 11.2). Chief among the differences are the inclusion in care management of cases according to the likelihood of future resource utilization rather than disease or diagnosis; consideration of but not reliance on clinical guidelines in care management; and care management's ability to address comorbidities in the Status One population.

Table 11.2. Care Management and Disease Management.

Care Management	Disease Management
Transcends conditions and ages	Disease-specific
Economic model—inclusion by risk of future complexity and high costs	Clinical model—inclusion by diagnosis
Guidelines useful but not essential	Guidelines relied on
Population-based predictive registries essential	Registries useful but not essential
Addresses comorbidities	Designed for the "average," singly diseased patient
Population-based economic and functional status measures	Outcomes often estimated; substituted intermediate clinical markers not relevant to leaders

Metrics and Outcomes

Disease management in its current incarnation offers few metrics that are useful and understandable to clinical and administrative leaders. Some programs are assessed in public health terms of dollars per year of life saved. Others are evaluated by the percentage decrease in some untoward outcome—for example, the percentage decrease in myocardial infarctions after so many years of the administration of HMG-CoA-class lipid-lowering agents. Still others may track ER visits, thirty- and sixty-day hospital readmissions, or five-year cancer-survival rates. Compendiums exist of hundreds of such measures, many of which have been suggested as clinical quality measures for disease management initiatives (Bowling, 1995).

All these measures miss important elements of the time frames peculiar to contemporary managed care. The principal time frame in a cost-driven marketplace is no more than one year, which corresponds to commercial contracting periods and the planning cycles of MCOs. Longer time frames are of considerable medical interest but are far more abstract to insurers and health care leaders. Members turn over at rates of 10 to 15 percent per year. Compliance with long-term drug therapies for asymptotic persons, as is the case with antihypertension and hypocholesterolemic agents, makes impacts on long-term outcomes that much more remote. Further, it is costly to gather data often existing only in paper medical records or financial records.

Some readers may find the one-year horizon for realizing cost savings to be myopic, but it is dictated by market conditions. Commercial payers define the managed care marketplace, and they are purchasing health care services chiefly on the basis of price. NCQA and HEDIS notwithstanding, price competition prevails. To pursue high-risk population health management while carefully selecting disease management programs on the basis of economic reality is a successful marketplace strategy.

Phasing out disease management programs that do not contribute to near-term cost efficiencies is not a heartless policy that consigns members to health care purgatory. There is every reason to believe that in the absence of disease management programs the clinical care rendered by credentialed professionals is in line with community standards, in a manner similar to FFS care.

Chapter Eight derived a set of economic and functional status outcome measures for population health management. These are suitable metrics for Status One patients and for all disease management programs. Such measures are monthly cross-sectional prevalence values. Outcome measures for specific disease management programs may include outcome measures peculiar to each disease process, but they should be derived from readily accessible data and minimize reliance on cumbersome chart reviews.

Case Example 11.1. Euglycemic Control of Diabetes Mellitus

Diabetes mellitus is a major morbidity and cost element in all managed care populations. National clinical trials (Diabetes Control and Complications Trial Research Group, 1993, 1996) have revealed that more frequent measurement and insulin dosing of diabetics can reduce kidney, eye, heart, and blood-vessel complications as soon as seven years after therapy is begun and may improve quality of life even sooner (Testa and Simonson, 1998). Most clinicians and their patients find the rigorous treatment schedules a challenge. Guidelines simplifying complex treatment protocols were designed for the Park Nicollet Clinic in Minnesota and subsequently offered to other practices for adoption (Mazze, Strock, Etzweiller, and Simonson, 1997). Outcome measures are patients' adherence to self-monitoring regimens and use of supporting materials. Hemoglobin A_1Cs are sampled as clinical markers for euglycemia (normal blood glucose values).

Strategies for educating clinicians and providing a variety of supporting materials to them constitute one type of disease management. The diabetes guidelines frequently increase patient autonomy in monitoring blood glucose levels and empower nurses through standing orders to make adjustments in insulin doses within agreed-on ranges. Diabetes is unusual among chronic conditions because daily glucose measurement is frequent, relevant to long-term outcomes, and amenable to statistical control charting and increased patient responsibility.

Another strategy is to create a specialty service within the delivery system. These "carve-ins" have been pursued for diabetes care, lipid-control clinics, and anticoagulation monitoring.

High-risk population health management for diabetics challenges programs focused on diabetes mellitus as a single disease. Typically, diabetic Status One patients are afflicted with other serious diseases and social-support challenges, which place them outside guidelines suited to the average patient. Recall Kenny Franco, the case example from Chapter Three, whose barriers to starting insulin therapy were social isolation and subclinical depression. These are essential issues that have to be resolved if we expect to affect the outcome for Kenny.

Case Example 11.2. Congestive Heart Failure

CHF disease management (Pezella, O'Mara, and Donahue, 1997) can use a carve-out strategy, where one or more services supplementing the usual clinical care are offered externally to the health care delivery system (Rich and Freedland, 1988; Rich and others, 1993; Rich and others, 1995; Rich and Beckman, 1996). In-home monitoring of patients with CHF and advanced-stage angina pectoris has been provided on a contractual basis to managed care organizations that do not offer such services themselves. Guidelines for related issues such as water and salt intake, diuretic use, and even in-home administration of intravenous inotropic agents are bundled together with the nursing services. Outcomes include hospital readmissions and patient satisfaction.

Challenges for Disease Management Programs

Wholesale adoption of disease management programs faces four important challenges (Holdford, 1996; Scott, 1995). First, often, as in the case example of the "tight control" of diabetes, a timing mismatch exists between clinical efforts and desired outcome (Diabetes Control and Complications Trial Study Group, 1995, 1998). More staff, more monitoring, and more medications are involved in tight control now, while benefits are years away. Given the rate of membership turnover, many of those consuming more intensive services now will not be served by the organization years hence. Second, single-disease programs generally do not benefit the comorbid Status One patient. The patients who will be generating the most medical costs are not the primary beneficiaries of disease management programs. Third, benefits Status One patients derive in the near term are not specific to the disease but rather are the result of how patients proactively manage their multiple diseases and social situation. Fourth, some MCOs distrust disease management programs associated with drug companies. Those programs administered by sales representatives and run by marketing departments do nothing to quash such suspicions.

Managed Care Strategic Considerations

When choosing which disease management programs to pursue, MCOs have these additional implications to consider beyond the priorities identified by population health analysis:

Adverse selection

Moral hazard

Diffusion of effort

Fragmentation of care

Burden to providers

Masquerade for formulary compliance or concurrent review

Contradictions among strategies

It is one thing to optimize the care of the acutely and chronically ill members once they are in an MCO; it is financially suicidal to attract them until capitation risk adjusters are further along than they are today. Short of advertising, organizations taking on large disease management staffs pose a moral hazard. They increase their operating costs over their competition without the bottom-line impacts to justify the increase. Many disease management programs, especially those involving "carve-out" services, can fragment the provision of care and confuse providers (Kurowski, 1998). Those sponsored by external organizations must be held accountable for pursuing the goals of the MCO.

The Future of Disease Management

Disease management programs can have a bright future in managed care. It is a future of fewer programs, targeted by economic segmentation of the population and each patient's clinical conditions. It is expected that many disease management vendors will consolidate around those that have compelling business models and that offer near-term savings. An incremental medical management strategy that stratifies members by financial and clinical risks and incrementally improves care for additional subgroups as resources allow will lead to financial success in the present and will seize the quality- and cost-conscious future of managed care.

Public policies that lead to slower membership turnover (for example, single-payer health-purchasing cooperatives or exclusive-provider networks) will encourage a longer-term focus. Multiyear premium pricing strategies will provide an increasingly solid economic basis for clinical improvements with longer and longer payback periods. Such strategies will catalyze the next round of systemwide improvements in quality throughout health care.

Although disease management programs have become popular, high-risk population health management should be afforded precedence in health organizations retaining financial risk. After the process of care has been made optimal for Status One patients, disease management programs should be introduced vigorously for those presenting a relatively more moderate clinical and financial risk. As care for these risk groups is optimized, additional efforts should then be made with patients at relatively lower risk of incurring future costs and experiencing clinical problems. This incremental process provides health care with a pathway to clinical excellence.

· · · · · · ·

In this chapter the deficiencies of disease management programs for use in high-risk population health care were considered. Among these deficiencies is the limited applicability of clinical guidelines given the comorbidities and unique social issues of the highest-risk patients. Redesigning care to meet the needs of Status One patients is an important step prior to embarking on disease management programs. When disease programs are considered, they should be chosen on the basis of their ability to extend benefits of care management to the frailest members and then to successive groups identified by future health and economic risk.

12

. . . .

Agenda for the Future

Researchers, clinicians, and administrators express considerable interest in acquiring the ability to predict high-utilizing patients and to constructively intervene with them. Because high-risk population health management is a new paradigm working across diagnoses, relatively little formal research has been done on its underpinnings or its most effective initiatives. This chapter surveys the backlog of issues awaiting evaluative research projects.

Leadership Decision Making and Proof of Efficacy

The challenge for managed care leaders is to improve the care of their neediest and costliest members with programs that have a strong empirical track record; they need to meet this challenge while being minimally encumbered by a slow and costly quasi-research infrastructure. The lean managed care operational environment does not foster long-term thinking or encourage academic depth. But the research questions asked here are important. They await funding and organizations willing to host clinical research.

The challenge for health care leaders is to advocate action now and to pursue in parallel funded research to address important long-term considerations. The threshold for business decision making has already been crossed by high-risk population health management for Status One patients, including near-term quality and cost impacts (Leveille and others, 1998; Forman, Kelliher, and Wood, 1997).

Proposals for Research

The high-risk population approach to care management discussed here raises a number of important questions. Formal research will be fruitful in a number of areas; funding formal protocols for researching these issues is a promising field for sponsorship by health services research organizations.

Many good studies that predict high use exist for particular diseases, including CHF, psychoses, and asthma. Studies predicting utilization across a general population are rarer. Health services research into reorganizing care for high-risk patients from a general population is even more unusual.

Standardize Outcomes

Research in the area of high-risk population health management must include metrics that not only are statistically and conceptually sound but also meet the needs of managed care leaders. They should include economic measures important to MCOs, and it should be expected that some level of improvement will be demonstrated in less than one year. For example, a study might be pursued on the impact of a new treatment for severe diabetics. In addition to the usual clinical measures—mortality rates, morbidity measures, laboratory tests—one-year PMPM costs and hospital utilization should also be measured.

Standardize the Research Population

The success of predictive modeling depends on the age structure of the population and the underlying prevalence of numerous diseases. To the extent that researchers employ various convenience samples and populations, results may not be comparable to those obtained in studies of a single disease.

The solution is to apply various predictive approaches to a single data set. HCFA researchers utilize a 10 percent random sample of Medicare claims and make it freely available to geriatric researchers. A comparable database for population health management would contain at least two years of demographics (omitting personal identifiers), claims, pharmacy data, and perhaps laboratory data on several hundred thousand people covered by managed care in representative major markets in each part of the country. The database would contain electronically accessible information and, therefore, would mirror the experience of likely users. The federal government or a private trade organization could construct and oversee use of such an important database.

Improve Predictive Models

An area of interest is improving the means of anticipating clinically complex patients on a population basis. We have already discussed applications of empirically derived trigger algorithms from leading and lagging indicators. Chapter Fourteen discusses the application of multiple linear and nonlinear regressions and artificial intelligence to this issue.

Determining the data that are the most valuable for stratifying managed care populations is an important collateral arena. Ascertaining the fewest possible pieces of relevant clinical information that will result in accurate models offers the promise of increasing precision and ease of application without expending effort to gather less valuable information.

Fruitful research has used various member questionnaires to obtain functional status assessments having some predictive value. A number of investigators quantify the predictive value of self-administered functional status tools in a general population. Their findings are extremely relevant to high-risk population health management. Combining such results with electronically accessible membership, claims, pharmacy, and laboratory data promises to improve the prognostic value of clinical registries. Combinations of questionnaires and electronically available data might be a power-ful boost to the ability to segment populations on the basis of future risk.

Many primary-care physicians and nurses believe at first that they can predict their high-risk patients better than any computer model can. Unfortunately, often half or more of their frail patients are not known to them for a variety of reasons. Conversely, providers are concerned about some patients who are not identified on computer-generated registries. This provider knowledge must be incorporated into any high-risk registry and serve as a basis for eval-uating and improving the computerized algorithms. Evaluation of provider-designated high-risk patients will reveal additional infor-mation about both approaches.

Assess Consumer Satisfaction

Little has been done to assess the satisfaction of intensely case man-aged patients and to compare it with the satisfaction of patients given usual kinds of care. In aggregate this type of research could suggest which initiatives are most welcomed by patients, thereby strengthening patient involvement and ownership.

Perform Cohort Analyses

Formal cohort analyses of Status One patients over long time peri-ods have not been done to date. Time-series results strongly suggest a marked financial impact associated with the aggressive care man-agement of these high-risk patients. Random, concurrent assign-ment within the same delivery system of at-risk patients paired with controls and consignment of outcomes into usual-care and care managed cells would eliminate some of the questions posed by the sequential time series.

Cohort analyses of the outcomes over time of patients in a single population served by the same provider system who are identified by algorithms, multiple-regression analyses, neural networks, and providers would yield additional information on the practicality of such predictive methods in clinical applications. The results would provide information over and above direct comparisons of registry size and would be sensitivity and predictive value positive (see Chapter Fourteen). They would reflect the ability of these various methods not only to predict costly patients but also to identify those whom clinicians can positively influence.

Delivery systems and HMOs seeking to improve their care of and financial results for high-risk patients should not proceed first on a research basis. Successful empirical approaches are known, and they are described in this book. Ad hoc, informal studies may not yield valid results, may detract from the important work of improving the process of care for frail members, and may delay and dilute expected financial gains.

Evaluate the Organization of Delivery Systems

Little formal research relates the organization of health care delivery for the high-risk population to outcomes meaningful to managed care leaders. An exception is research on a program for delivering health care to seniors in the Puget Sound area (Leveille and others, 1998); the results have been incorporated into care planning for Status One patients and the group internal medicine care pioneered by Kaiser Permanente in Colorado (Beck and others, 1997).

Several attributes of such research make it useful to managed care leaders. Interventions are on a population basis rather than for cherry-picked subsets or convenience samples. The interventions are clearly described and are implemented on a broad scale across the population. Results include outcome measures readily understandable to managed care practitioners—PMPM costs and savings, hospital utilization rates—all within a one-year time frame.

Measure the Effects of Information Systems

The communication of care plans, the provision of links to community resources, the enlistment of experts in the care planning process, and the involvement of patients electronically in their care plans are all new, promising fields in their infancy. Internet applications and tactics for the care of high-risk individuals and controlled measurement of the impact of such innovations are fertile areas for medical informatics research.

• • • • • • •

This chapter discussed several opportunities for research into optimal high-risk population health management. The possible areas for such research include standardizing a managed care research database, choosing inputs and outcomes relevant to managed care leaders, advancing the state of knowledge on high-risk predictive modeling, characterizing consumer satisfaction among the very ill, comparing modes of delivering care, and harnessing the emerging capabilities of intranets and IT.

Part IV

· ·

Sources and Rationale

13

Total Quality Management
Concepts, High-Risk Patient Customers, Measures, and Focus

In this chapter several tenets and practices of quality management are examined with respect to their application to high-risk population health management. The background of the quality movement, application of the Pareto principle, ways of identifying customer needs, and quality control metrics are discussed.

Clinical quality improvement concepts and strategies find their sources in industrial Total Quality Management (TQM) and the quality improvement field (Ishikawa, 1985). Readers may have some familiarity with the topic through the closely related Continuous Quality Improvement (CQI) and the outcomes research field. Excellent monographs are available on the application of quality management in medicine (Berwick, Godfrey, and Roessner, 1990; Goonan, 1995). For those unfamiliar with the quality movement and its applications in medicine, a critical discussion of its origins and contemporary utility for high-risk population health management follows.

Briefly stated, CQI asserts that any product or service can be improved to world-class levels by defining quality on the customer's terms, identifying the production process, and applying improvement methods and statistical techniques to systematically monitor the quality of the process and the resulting product.

Quality Management and the
Medical Scientific Method

The quality movement advocates major process changes on the basis of experience gained outside the laboratory and away from highly controlled experimental environments. Although the movement arose and has been used most extensively in manufacturing settings, advocates have enthusiastically adapted its methods to clinical situations—though not without controversy (Kassirer, 1993a).

Instituting major changes on the basis of a systematic approach to empirical practice is a departure from traditional ways of improving medical care. The ideal practice of clinical medicine has for decades been based on the execution of randomized, double-blind clinical trials for deciding optimal therapies. In the absence of such studies, wide variations were tolerated and remained unquantified for a long time (Wennberg, Freeman, and Culp, 1987). By contrast, advocates of CQI not only propagate best practices derived from formal medical research but also pursue local systematic improvements of any clinical and administrative processes important to quality. It is important to distinguish CQI from past practices, for adopting the tools of quality improvement will lead to changes in how medicine is practiced and improved, changes that randomized clinical trials could not foster.

The rigid experimental medical paradigm tends to conform to and reinforce the current state. Experimental clinical studies attempt to control for all variables. They are lengthy, complex, and costly. Sponsors of controlled clinical trials are far fewer than those who fund basic research and studies of drugs and devices. Peer reviewers of such research operate within the experimental paradigm and therefore tend to perpetuate and magnify the importance of such endeavors to the exclusion of empirical practice.

Both approaches to understanding opportunities for improvement are essential. Both approaches have an important role in population health management, particularly in areas where they are likely to yield positive and timely solutions. Processes of care for Status One patients are based on quality improvement theory and experience.

The door is open to a variety of controlled trials of methods of identifying high-risk patients, IT systems, and clinical intervention strategies (see Chapter Twelve). Such studies should be pursued, but organizations serious about improving care for frail and costly managed care members must act now in the face of economic imperatives. It does not take a randomized clinical trial to observe that current approaches to managed care have failed to fully meet the needs of high-risk patients.

A dramatic example of the paradigmatic contrast can be seen in the achievement of reducing postoperative mortality for cardiac revascularization surgery. A consortium of New England hospitals set up a team to map operative and supportive processes involved in the hospitalizations, surgery, and immediate recovery period for coronary bypass surgery. Quality improvements engendered by altering aspects of the processes thought to be important resulted in a 25 percent reduction in postoperative mortality (Melanka and O'Connor, 1995). Not only did the results far exceed the improvements expected from randomized clinical trials of single, isolated variables from among the myriad activities associated with coronary bypass and revascularization surgery, but the results were achieved with modest expense.

The fact that breakthrough outcomes resulted from using quality management techniques did not go unnoticed, with its implications for the field of clinical research and for peer review of what constitutes valid research (Melanka and O'Connor, 1998). The TQM methods of the Northern New England Cardiovascular Disease Study Group deviated greatly from the gold standard of double-blind, randomized clinical trials.

Customer Definition

The foundation of quality management is to identify the customers, quantify quality in their view, and improve it. Juran (1992) defines quality as fitness for use. Every valued product or service has a customer, and that customer defines quality and the standard for "fitness for use."

Who the customer is for health care is not obvious. W. Edwards Deming, the proponent of quality management credited with engendering brilliant successes in the postwar auto industry, said, "A suitable definition for quality of medical care is a perennial problem among administrators of medical care and people doing research in the subject. It seems simple to anyone [who] has not tried it" (1986, p. 171).

In American health care, the purchaser of health care is not the direct consumer (leaving aside the payment of deductibles and co-insurance). Business is the chief payer and customer for commercial managed care, as are the HCFA, which oversees Medicare managed care plans for the elderly, and state governments for Medicaid. Identifying the customer in the health care environment is more complex than identifying the customer in the automobile industry, an analogy often made by quality management gurus. For Toyota, Ford, or Daimler Benz-Chrysler the customers are consumers who decide whether the automobile they purchased meets or exceeds the performance expected of a vehicle in its class. If we apply practices in health care to the automobile analogy, it is as if the consumer's employer is the buyer, but the consumer gets to choose the type of auto and to use it. It is not surprising that under FFS medicine, most patients gravitated toward the Mercedes Benz and the Ferrari. The growth of managed care can be seen as the result of business and government payers assessing the cost of the health care purchases made on behalf of their employees and citizens.

The chief customer of high-risk population health management, and indeed of all managed care, is the payer. Patients are consumers of health services and undoubtedly benefit from efforts to increase their functional status. Yet it would be disingenuous to characterize population health management as something other than a strategy to redesign the care for frail and unstable patients for the purpose of overall efficiency. Cost savings from high-risk population health management contribute more to increased efficiency in delivering services in the managed care environment than any strategy yet conceived. Savings can be used to lower premiums, add to reserves, or increase profits.

The NCQA (Skolnick, 1997) has stimulated a renewed focus on clinical quality, but those familiar with the health care marketplace know that price competition dominates (Prager, 1998). Organizations thriving in the current environment will produce the Toyotas and Fords of health care, moderately priced and with good value (as indicated by the quality-to-price ratio). Consumers may still want the luxury versions, but the true customers are not buying. MCOs that master the current environment—and high-risk population health management, starting with Status One patients—possess the skills and structure to extend this strategy to larger and larger parts of their membership on the basis of economic risk. They will be in position to seize the future beyond price competition.

Medical and nursing audiences often balk at the assertion that health care customers define quality and protest that their patients and clients are not customers. They believe that state licensing boards, specialty societies, the American Medical Association, the American Nursing Association, specialty examining boards, or any number of accrediting agencies define quality. The quality movement asserts that such societies, boards, and associations serve the purpose of verifying education and competencies, yet the ultimate arbiter of quality is the customer who purchases the service.

Quality by Inspection Versus Conformance to Customer-Oriented Specifications

Quality management is philosophically opposed to reliance on inspection. Instead it advocates optimizing the process by identifying its critical components and determining and improving specifications for each one. Specifications are linked to the customer's view of quality, and each worker is responsible for meeting them. High-risk population health management focuses on the processes of identification, assessment, and care of frail and unstable managed care members rather than erecting "inspection" barriers to services that their health care providers feel are needed.

The issue is even more important in health care than in manufacturing. Service errors cannot be corrected in the same way that a defective physical object can be repaired. Nevertheless, total reliance on inspection is rife in managed care. It is the norm for MCOs with delegated risk to preauthorize all inpatient care, home-care services, and prescriptions for certain drugs. Much of medical management in managed care is based on 100 percent inspection only. It casts an entire and costly infrastructure in the role of quality inspectors who second-guess clinician recommendations. Physicians having their decisions reviewed in this manner feel as devalued as the lowest ranking Detroit assembly worker did prior to the transformation of that industry by quality management.

In fairness, in some situations total reliance on inspection may be justified: when the cost of a missed defect is so catastrophic that the cost of inspecting each item is justified. Most would agree that inspecting each and every fuel-tank O-ring in NASA space shuttles is justified, considering the consequences that component's failure inflicted on the shuttle *Challenger's* crew during its catastrophic take-off in 1986. The consequences of a missed inpatient authorization are far different and more benign, a hospital stay that may or may not be as long as the normative standard being employed.

Decision trees provide leaders with a disciplined approach to deciding whether total inspection justifies the cost. An example would be measuring the cost-benefit of an HMO preauthorization process. Inputs include the percentage of cases that "inspection" culls out (not including those decisions reversed by appeals processes), the cost of alternative care, the cost of inpatient care had the preauthorizations not taken place, the population size, the expected number of admissions, and the size and overall costs of required staff. A complete analysis would also factor in the cost of software and equipment needed to gather and process authorization data. Although preauthorization inspectors detect and cull out a significant dollar amount of avoidable inpatient admissions, the overall return on investment may be far less. Decision analyses lend themselves to sensitivity analyses—that is, determining the threshold of factors that would justify the effort.

A drawback to these economic analyses is the requirement of assigning a dollar value to each factor. Putting a dollar value on the clinicians' view of precertifications is difficult, yet it is quite significant. Organized medicine labels such practices in managed care the *hassle factor*, which is the cause of increasing rancor. Such strategies may have some value in an FFS environment but can be unnecessary where providers are accustomed to moderately or aggressively managed inpatient utilization.

In some cases the cost of staffs dedicated to utilization management and utilization review do not warrant their existence. In such a situation, resources may be better directed toward population health management and facilitating the care of Status One patients.

Tools for Statistical Process Control

Once a process for producing a good or service is defined, intermediate processes can be defined, each with identifiable customers and suppliers, inputs and outputs, and the potential to specify customer requirements. Once these intermediate processes are defined, critical steps can be analyzed and systematically improved. TQM methods for Statistical Process Control (SPC) constitute a toolbox that can be used to identify and break down process barriers that impair quality.

The steps for any process that produces a good or service can be identified with final or intermediate customers and suppliers. Typically a cross-functional team will collaborate in order to document the steps involved in a complex process. The *cause-and-effect diagram* is a tool to facilitate discussion and to sort out potential causes of quality problems. These fish-bone, or Ishikawa, charts provide structure for discussing a process and its vulnerable points. "Bones" on the chart typically include personnel, materials, methods, and equipment. Quality will have been defined a priori according to customer specifications.

Pareto diagrams identify key problems or symptoms that impair a quality outcome. The premise is that a small number of faults cause the majority of malfunctions. As Juran (1988, pp. 27–29) put it, focusing improvement efforts requires "separating the vital few from the useful many." The Pareto principle asserts that 80 percent of defects are caused by a manageable 20 percent of the range of possible causes. Quality management advocates full concentration on the 20 percent of causes until they are greatly improved and then incrementally proceeding to the remaining causes of impaired quality in the order of their contribution to the problem. *Histograms* are a means of further teasing out causes and effects of quality lapses. *Check sheets*, *scatter diagrams*, and *stratification* are methods of empirically testing and optimizing the variables identified in the cause-and-effect and Pareto processes.

Control charts set statistical limits for the few critical variables, detecting special causes of variation so that they can be eliminated. Points outside control limits, typically three standard deviations from the mean value in manufacturing and two standard deviations from the mean value in health care, indicate a special cause, which can be identified. Meanwhile, quality improvement efforts focus on common problems that, when improved, will shift the overall process capability and in doing so will increase overall quality.

Applications in clinical practice often seem to be not as straightforward as those in industry. Cycle times for ultimate clinical effect can be long. Outcomes for innovations in cancer care are five- and ten-year survival rates. The focus often switches to intermediate outcomes, such as glycosylated hemoglobin levels in diabetics, when the ultimate clinical outcomes are the absence or presence of cardiovascular, optical, neurological, and renal problems years in the future. Unlike the gauging of industrial processes, even with intermediate outcomes long periods often ensue between clinical measurements, or excessive effort is necessary in order to obtain quantitative measures from chart reviews.

Using a Pareto Diagram to Analyze Diagnoses

A frequent approach to clinical improvement is to stratify a population by diagnoses and to concentrate efforts on the "vital few." In a Pareto diagram of principal diagnoses of Status One patients (as judged by the treating clinicians), no one diagnosis predominates (see Figure 13.1 and Table 13.1). The most common single diagnosis is coronary atherosclerosis, but it accounts for less than 6 percent of the total. Although exact percentages are a reflection of the demographics and risk profile of the underlying population, 11 percent seniors in the example cited here, the observation is particularly robust: the largest single category among Status One patients' chief diagnoses is "all other." No single disease initiative or combination of them could possibly have an impact on the entire group. Further, the Pareto chart does not reflect the frequent comorbidities and social complexities among these patients, as previously described.

One response to the conundrum is to roll up diagnoses into Diagnostic Related Groups or into even broader categories. The

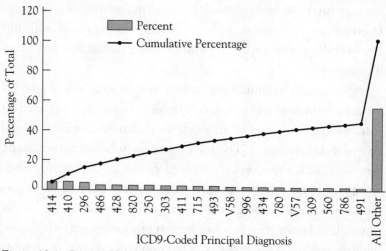

Figure 13.1. Pareto Chart of Principal Diagnoses of Status One Patients
N = 1,509 patients encountered among 100,000 in the course of a year.
Data from Forman, Kelliher, and Wood (1997).

result is typically to identify cardiovascular diseases as the chief clinical cause of high costs and high complexity. Unfortunately, such a tack has little operational meaning. Rolling up myocardial infarction, CHF, cardiac arrhythmia, angina pectoris, and myriad other diagnoses into one category may force-fit a round Pareto bar into a square quality management hole, but it has no meaning for those designing practical clinical interventions that will produce near-term efficiencies and improved functional status.

Setting Quality Standards

Since the late 1980s payers have increasingly asserted their interest in obtaining value for health care expenditures. Despite words to the contrary, MCOs currently compete almost exclusively on price and network. Quality may become a distinguishing factor in the future, but it is not currently (Greene, 1998a; Larkin, 1997).

The NCQA is an industry-backed organization whose HEDIS is the data set by which commercial payers judge MCO quality.

Table 13.1. Principal Diagnoses of Status One Patients.

ICD9 Code	Description	Percentage of Cases	Cumulative Percentage
414	Coronary atherosclerosis	5.10	5.10
410	Acute myocardial infarction	4.92	10.02
296	Affective psychosis	4.37	14.39
486	Pneumonia	2.67	17.06
428	Congestive heart failure	2.55	19.61
820	Femoral fracture	2.55	22.16
250	Diabetes with complications	2.43	24.59
303	Alcohol dependence	2.13	26.72
411	Coronary artery disease without occlusion	2.13	28.85
715	Osteoarthritis	1.94	30.79
493	Asthma	1.82	32.61
V58	Chemotherapy and aftercare	1.70	34.31
996	Device complications	1.64	35.95
434	Cerebral vascular accident	1.52	37.47
780	Syncope; coma	1.46	38.93
V57	Rehabilitation	1.34	40.27
309	Adjustment reaction	1.15	41.42
560	Intestinal obstruction	1.15	42.57
786	Chest pain, noncardiac	1.15	43.72
491	Bronchitis	1.09	44.81
All other		55.19	100.00

Note: Chief diagnoses for acutely and chronically ill patients during 1995 baseline year. $N = 1,509$.

Source: Forman, S. A., Kelliher, M., and Wood, G. "Clinical Improvement with Bottom-Line Impact: Custom Care Planning for Patients with Acute and Chronic Illnesses in a Managed Care Setting." American Journal of Managed Care, 1997, 3(7), 1039–1048; by permission.

Reflecting its business roots, the NCQA incorporates quality management principles in its accreditation requirements, which are as follows:

Defined workflows and measures for all key processes including medical management

Ownership and accountability for all key processes

Demonstrated, objective improvement in key processes

Ongoing improvement and corrective actions

NCQA assessment of clinical quality is in its infancy (Prager, 1998). Initial HEDIS versions focus on preventive services such as mammography and immunizations more for the ready availability of data and recognized national standards of care than for the importance of these issues to overall system costs. Assessment of clinical quality across organizations is hampered by the inaccessibility of clinical markers and end points, which are often maintained in hard copy and protected by strict confidentiality practices. A sampling of successful quality improvement efforts in MCOs, especially the growing IPAs, reveals programs that avoid data-inaccessibility issues and whose results have short measurement cycles.

Another challenge relates to the accountability of HMO plans for HEDIS clinical measures. The HMOs envision differentiating among themselves in the future marketplace by competing on clinical quality. However, health care delivery systems typically contract with more than one HMO. There is no reason to believe that clinical practices for one insurer's patients are essentially different from those for another's patients when the care is rendered by a delivery system serving multiple insurers, and providers rarely know their patient's health plan.

Most current clinical quality improvement initiatives do not change the processes of care in any fundamental way. Table 13.2 is a sampling of IPA clinical quality improvement initiatives capable of showing quantifiable outcomes. None would be expected to contribute to the bottom line of overall health care costs. Most employ administrative data sets, obviating the need for costly and cumbersome chart reviews for extracting clinical end points.

Table 13.2. Sampling of Independent Practice Association Clinical-
Improvement Initiatives.

Initiative	Intervention	End Point	Data Sources
Reduce Cesarean rate	Targeted education for vaginal birth after Cesarean	Cesarean section	Administrative claims
Improve asthma care	Distribute peak expiratory flow meters and encourage inhaled steroids	Asthma ER and hospitalizations	Adminstrative claims: ER and pharmacy
Improve immunization rates	Mailings	Immunizations	Administrative claims
Increase mammography rate	Mailings	Mammograms	Administrative claims
Improve diabetes care	Provider and patient reminders	Glycosylated hemoglobin, retinal exams, foot exams	Chart audits

The Foundation for Accountability (FACCT) promotes an evolving set of quality standards extending to FFS medicine and including additional consumer representation. Because it lacks a direct link to payers, its development has been slower than for the NCQA HEDIS measures, which enjoy the sponsorship of business health coalitions and which could become important in future purchasing decisions.

The Baldrige Award is conferred by the U.S. Department of Commerce to encourage, as a matter of international competitiveness, the adoption of quality principles in business and to recognize organizations particularly successful at it. A division specifically for health care organizations has been introduced. Perversely, organizations investing extensively in quality at the current time, especially if they do not broadly approach the expensive Status One population, impose a cost disadvantage on themselves against minimalist competitors.

Quality programs have acquired a mixed reputation in the health sector in large part because of their application in hospital downsizing and reengineering. Additionally, although quality improvement teams have provided an important forum within organizations for discussing current processes, results have been viewed as insignificant. High-risk population health management, by focusing improvement efforts on the near-term, intends to reverse that perception.

Metrics

Choice of metrics is a reflection of quality in the customer's view. The customers for population health management initiatives aimed at improving Status One patient care are leaders of risk-bearing MCOs and payers. Metrics, as discussed in Chapter Eight, reflect payer concerns. Included are utilization rates and PMPM costs as well as process measures needed to lead the effort. For Status One patients, their own global view of their health, as extracted from functional status instruments, is the main clinical outcome measure. Measures made on behalf of other stakeholders—health services researchers, for example—are not recommended unless funded and energized by dedicated resources.

Focus

Quality is improved by concentrating on the few issues revealed by Pareto charting to be the greatest barriers to improvement. Pareto charting of the highest-risk Status One patients reveals that the challenge is to improve the care of "all others" rather than those with particular diseases. Clinical leaders can be diverted by the tendency to tackle many issues; they often lack a clear idea of which are the "vital few."

Often, leaders in health care hail the sheer volume of projects and improvement teams initiated. Instead, it is success, more specifically results, with the critical few issues that makes a difference.

Population health management should start with Status One patients by virtue of their small numbers, clinical instability, and disproportionately large financial impact. Prime areas for improvement efforts included removing barriers to accessing care and optimizing the content of clinical care.

· · · · · · · ·

In this chapter aspects of CQI were discussed in relation to molding population health management. The Pareto principle demonstrates that Status One patients, rather than those with specific diseases, make up the most attractive population segment to begin clinical quality initiatives. The organized clinical quality movement has so far contributed little to managing high-risk, high-cost patients. Nevertheless, from a quality management standpoint, achieving robust processes and clinical services for Status One patients is amply justified by customer needs and marketplace realities.

Epidemiology

Power and Limits of Statistical Approaches

T his chapter addresses what leaders need to know of the epidemiological foundations of population health management
(Rothman, 1998; Kleinbaum, Kupper, and Morgenstern, 1982).
Topics include a definition of populations, the mathematical tools
available for quantifying the accuracy of tests, more advanced methods of segmenting the population, and essential accuracy measures
for registries of Status One and chronic disease patients. A working
knowledge of these concepts will empower leaders to get actionable
and meaningful information from their own staffs and from vendors,
and to hold their own organizations accountable for true, bottom-
line results.

Thus far the accuracy of tools to identify high-risk patients has
been assumed. In fact, the task of generating accurate registries of
high-risk patients is a complex one. In this chapter, we will come
to a common understanding of the epidemiology behind population
health management and its current capabilities for prospectively
identifying frail and costly patients.

Understanding the Population

Population health management begins with segmenting a group of
people according to their needs. In managed care, the population

is a group of people who obtain their health care under a defined set of benefits.

Commercial HMO members have most of their medical premiums paid for by employers. The population comprises employed people and family members who have a particular prepaid health plan. Another population contains senior Medicare risk members. Many states have prepaid Medicaid plans that define a population of covered members with demographic, income, and disease characteristics distinct from those of commercial and senior managed care members. From the perspective of the risk-bearing provider group, total managed care membership comprises senior, commercial, and Medicaid subgroups.

HMOs cannot set their premiums unless they know the attributes of their members and can project future utilization and costs. Currently, interest is heightened by the common practice of setting HMO premium rates competitively and risk-rating employee groups. As provider groups increasingly take on financial risk, they need a working knowledge of population-based metrics. The movement toward improving quality in HMOs also depends heavily on the ability of managed care to quantify its population subgroups. Table 14.1 summarizes population boundaries from the perspective of organizations involved in health care.

When considering quantitative measures in the managed care environment, it is important to focus on the appropriate population and to be sure that outcome measures are drawn from the same group. Epidemiologists refer to the need for valid rates as "making sure the numerator and denominator come from the same place." To err on this leads to aberrant data and faulty conclusions.

Incidence and Prevalence

A step on the road to segmenting a managed care population is to understand expressions for characterizing new cases of a health condition and the total burden of that condition. The rate of a newly

Table 14.1. Prepaid-Member Populations from the Perspective of Health-Related Organizations.

Organization	Population
HMO	Eligible members and dependents ("covered lives" taken together) paying premiums
Group practice, medical services organization, PHO, or PPM	Managed care members with full or shared risk to the provider organization
Self-insured employer	Participating employees, dependents, some retirees
Medicaid	Participating families, subject to state-mandated income limits
Public health department and hospital charity care	Uninsured population on a geographical basis. Further divisions if involved in Medicaid

diagnosed disease or condition occurring during a time period is an *incidence* rate. *Prevalence* is the total number of cases present during that time (period prevalence, or at a particular instant in time—point prevalence). A simple relationship exists between incidence and prevalence in a stable group. Prevalence is equal to the product of incidence multiplied by the average duration of the condition. In this equation any two figures permit the calculation of the third.

$$P = I \times D_{average}$$

where

P = prevalence, units are cases or people

I = incidence, units are cases or people over time

D = average duration of the condition among all cases, in time units

. . . .

Case Example 14.1. Diabetes Incidence and Prevalence in a Group Practice

Consider the case of estimating patients with adult-onset diabetes in a group practice from epidemiological information. Once diagnosed, each patient will be a diabetic for life. Diabetics cared for by one group of physicians may live twenty years on average following diagnosis. In line with American Diabetes Association findings for all Americans, at least 5 percent of the patients in a family practice are expected to be diagnosed diabetics. Yet few new diagnoses will be made. These are incident cases. And few will die or leave each month. In a steady state environment, the number of diabetics in a clinical practice remains constant, the newly diagnosed patients replacing those afflicted with the condition who leave the practice or pass away. A registry of all diabetic people is a *prevalence*. In a group practice, if the incidence of newly diagnosed diabetics is low, say four people a month, while twenty years is the average duration, then prevalence can be calculated in this way:

$$P = I \times D_{average}$$
$$P = 4 \text{ patients/month} \times 20 \text{ years} \times 12 \text{ months/year}$$
$$P = 960 \text{ patients}$$

. . . .

It is useful to categorize commonly used managed care statistics as incidence or prevalence measures. Typical incidence measures include these:

Newly diagnosed disease cases

Membership turnover per year

Dollars spent for a group of people over a year

Inpatient admissions per thousand members per month

$PMPM

Some typical prevalence statistics are these:

Disease registries of current members

Current members of a particular health plan

Everyone with a disease at a given point in time; for example, 0.5 to 1.0 percent of a membership are Status One patients

Inpatient hospital days per thousand members per month

Inpatient census

By categorizing statistics in this way, leaders can derive important characteristics about the population they serve and design initiatives targeted to their particular needs. Inpatient admission rate per thousand (admits), inpatient days per thousand, and length of stay are, respectively, incidence, prevalence, and duration statistics. Status One and chronic disease registries are a form of prevalence, while the rate at which new members join or leave the registries is an incidence statistic.

Quantifying the Accuracy of Tests Identifying At-Risk People

The effectiveness of high-risk population case management depends on identifying members in most need and aggressively managing their care. Predictive models that identify too many people not truly at high risk will dissipate efforts and dilute results. In Chapter Nine, the theory of what constituted high-risk cases was given an empirical treatment culminating in the registry size and the $PMPY for varied approaches applied to the same managed care population. Epidemiology permits greater precision in describing the accuracy of a method to proactively identify high-cost and high clinical complexity cases. After defining a few epidemiological measures here, we present the four essential characteristics for describing a predictive model's accuracy.

The idea of accuracy must be further teased out to have meaning in the context of characterizing population-segmentation and diagnostic procedures. Is an accurate model one that identifies all the diseased people we are concerned about and extraneous cases as well? Or is an accurate model one in which there is absolute certainty of the condition at the expense of missing cases? If the test model is negative, just how much certainty is there that the condition is not in fact there?

Whether arranging for mammography screening for the early detection of breast cancer, identifying undiagnosed diabetics by serum blood testing at routine physical examinations, or stratifying a managed care population to identify high-risk patients, health care professionals must have a precise means of describing accuracy. Clarifying the degree of accuracy on several measures enables us to interpret our findings and to design interventions to suit patients' needs and the capabilities of our tools and methods.

Accuracy means different things in different contexts. A false-positive urine screen done in the workplace to ascertain drug abuse is very different from a false-positive screen for sickle cell anemia. With urine screens false positives are less tolerated because considerable social condemnation comes with illicit drug use, and there is only a small hope of therapeutic intervention in randomly identified drug abusers. With screens for sickle cell anemia, false positives are better tolerated because African Americans usually want to know whether they carry the sickle-cell trait for family-planning purposes, and accurate confirmatory tests are readily available. In the case of colon cancer, clinicians accept a large number of false-positive stool samples for occult blood because the desire to identify people at an early stage, when the disease is most treatable, outweighs the inconvenience of having a false-positive test.

Accuracy measures of all sorts depend on the ability of a test to distinguish people with a real disease or condition from people who do not have it. Absolute knowledge of the condition is assumed in order to compare test methods. Short of death or the pathologist's

diagnosis from microscopic examination of fixed laboratory speci-
mens, there is always some controversy about the selection of the
standard against which we compare. Usually some widely accepted
diagnostic process is identified as the "consensus standard," or "gold
standard," against which any new approaches are compared. For
example, screening and diagnostic procedures for detecting coronary atherosclerotic heart disease can be compared by using
angiograms to distinguish between evident coronary arterial nar-
rowing and plaques. Cardiologists and radiologists tell us that these
methods have some small error, but for purposes of discussion and
comparison coronary arteriography is accepted as the consensus
standard.

Accuracy Measures and Two-by-Two Tables

In order for a test's performance to be quantified, it must be empirically determined in a known population. A two-by-two table is
widely used by epidemiologists to break out the components of test
accuracy. As shown in Figure 14.1 the two attributes are stated as
either present or absent. One axis is the presence or absence of the
attribute according to the consensus standard, while the other axis
is presence or absence of the condition using the test method. The
two dichotomous variables break the population N into four
subgroups—a, b, c, and d.

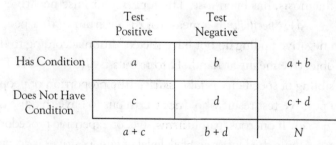

	Test Positive	Test Negative	
Has Condition	a	b	$a + b$
Does Not Have Condition	c	d	$c + d$
	$a + c$	$b + d$	N

Figure 14.1. Two-by-Two Table: Epidemiological Definitions.

A handy attribute of the two-by-two table is that all nine values, four in the table and five marginal sums, can be calculated by simple arithmetic from any combination of four values.

All people who unequivocally have the condition according to the consensus standard are designated $a + b$. This value must be known in advance in a research database to derive the other values. Conversely, everyone who absolutely does not have the disease or condition according to the consensus standard is designated $c + d$. People who show up positive by the test or screening method and do have the disease according to the consensus standard are included in a. Those who unequivocally have the condition but test negative are b. Similarly, some people can test positive for the disease or condition but not, in fact, have it (c). The remainder are those neither testing positive nor having the disease or condition (d). Everyone testing positive, regardless of whether they truly are afflicted, are captured by $a + c$. All testing negative, regardless of whether they truly have the disease or condition, are found in $b + d$.

With this groundwork, one is now ready to define the components of accuracy that health care leaders need to know. Refer to Figure 14.1 again. *Sensitivity* is the proportion of people who test positive and who truly have the condition. The sensitivity value can by calculated by $a/(a + b)$. The twin of sensitivity is the proportion of *false negatives*. These people truly have the condition but have a negative test. In this situation an opportunity to proceed with a variety of effective treatments, all of which work better with early diagnosis, has been lost. The formula for false negatives is $b/(b + d)$. *Specificity* is a measure of the certainty that people with a negative finding do not have the condition according to the most objective means at hand. The formula is $d/(c + d)$. The close sibling of specificity is *false positive*, the proportion of people with a positive test result who do not turn out to have the disease, $c/(a + c)$. If onerous, painful, invasive, or expensive procedures must occur, only the lowest possible level of false positives is acceptable. This is the case with AIDS blood testing and routine screen-ing of urine for abuse of drugs. The clinician and administrator eas-ily comprehend the predictive value of a positive test, $a/(a + c)$ or *predictive value positive*. Of all people with a positive test, it quan-tifies the portion who truly have the condition.

Case Example 14.2. Two or More Hospitalizations as a Predictor of High Utilization During the Following Year

Empirically derived data for a population of 100,000 reveal 1,250 high utilizers. Employing multiple hospitalizations as a high-risk population trigger will generate a registry of 900. Sensitivity is determined to be 11 percent, from which one calculates $a = 138$ (see Figure 14.2).

The remaining quantities can be determined by simple arithmetic from the four known quantities (see Figure 14.3).

	Trigger Positive	Trigger Negative	
Has Condition	$a = 138$	b	$a + b = 1{,}250$
Does Not Have Condition	c	d	$c + d$
	$a + c = 900$	$b + d$	$N = 100{,}000$

Figure 14.2. Known Values for Sample Calculation.

	Trigger Positive	Trigger Negative	
Has Condition	$a = 138$	$b = 1{,}112$	$a + b = 1{,}250$
Does Not Have Condition	$c = 762$	$d = 97{,}988$	$c + d = 98{,}750$
	$a + c = 900$	$b + d = 99{,}100$	$N = 100{,}000$

Figure 14.3. Completed Sample Calculation.

Predictive value positive = $a/(a + c)$ = 138/900 = 15.3 percent

False positive = $c/(a + c)$ = 762/900 = 84.7 percent

False negative = $b/(b + d)$ = 1,112/99,100 = 1.12 percent

Operating Characteristics of a Test

Precision of clinical tests in different groups of people is referred to as the operating characteristics of a test. Even when sensitivity and specificity have been determined correctly, the test will perform differently in a population according to the number of diseased people it contains.

Operating characteristics directly affect how useful screening diagnostic tests and questionnaires are in identifying needy people from a larger group. Operating characteristics are related to predictive value positive. The higher the prevalence of the condition or disease in the population, the higher the predictive value positive for any test characterized by a known sensitivity and specificity (see Figure 14.4). Conversely, when the disease or condition is rare in a population, it will yield a lower predictive value positive, even with the same test.

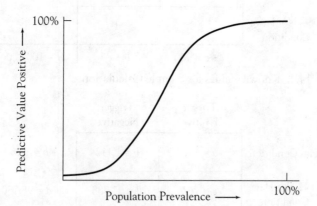

Figure 14.4. Operating Characteristics of a Test.

Methods of Sorting the High-Risk Population

The challenge in identifying Status One patients is that they are relatively rare in any population. Test procedures to identify them face the reality of unfavorable operating characteristics for any level of sensitivity or specificity. Chapter Three described a practical approach to overcoming this challenge, one based on computer modeling from leading and lagging indicators supplemented by patients added to the Status One registry on the basis of clinical judgment. A discussion follows of methods currently being applied to high-risk predictive modeling, so that the reader may become an intelligent customer of such work.

Multiple Regression

The purpose of regression methodologies is to measure the strength of the association between Y, called the dependent variable, and any number of X's, called the independent variables. A variety of electronically accessible data may be used as independent variables that predict economic outcomes in order to identify Status One patients. Because of the rigor of the assumptions needed to execute multiple regression analyses, the methodology has limited usefulness in population medical care management. There are many excellent texts on regression methodologies (Kleinbaum, 1997). The following discussion of multiple regression outcomes and assumptions will aid the managed care leader in becoming an informed initiator and consumer of such analyses.

Regression fits an equation to the dependent variables that are predictive of the outcome, or independent, variable. Nonlinear regressions for Status One patients take the form of equations whose independent variables have various coefficients, powers, and log transformations that together equal high medical expenses in a future period. The r^2 value, called the coefficient of determination, is a statistic describing how good the fit of the equation is for the dependent and independent variable. To measure how well a regression line fits the data, total variation among the dependent variables is divided into two parts—variation that can and cannot be explained by the regression line. The value of r^2 could quantify how much variation in cost, the Status One outcome measure, is explained by the regression equation. An r^2 value of 1.0 would mean that the regression is 100 percent accurate in correctly predicting the independent-variable outcome.

The correlation coefficient r may be more familiar to audiences who read medical journals and research articles. It measures how closely one value varies with another and ranges in value from -1 to $+1$. A value of 1 is a perfect relationship of variables changing in tandem; -1 describes an inverse relationship. Correlation coefficient r is the square root of the coefficient of determination, r^2.

Values of r^2 can be misused. A frequent error is to develop a high r^2 equation on a data set without testing only to find it a poor predictor in a subsequent situation. It is better to randomize data into a hypothesis generation set for equation development and fitting, holding data in reserve on which to test the equation. The r^2 to report would be the one arising from the test set, thereby simulating field conditions where it will be used.

Multiple regression assumptions are difficult to meet in the high-risk population, where disease-related information is regularly skewed one way or another or where the characteristics of the population are sometimes not fully known. In multiple regression, X and Y variables are assumed to be normally distributed random variables. The standard deviation of the independent Y is assumed to be constant for all values of X and the standard deviation of the X dependent variable is assumed to be constant for all values of Y. Y independent variables should not be correlated with one another; rather they are assumed to be independently linked to the X outcome variable. When atherosclerotic heart disease, for example, is a Y independent variable, it will in fact be correlated with other independent variables like age, sex, hypertension, hyperlipidemia, and diabetes. Such correlations among variables are described as multiple collinearity and conspire to limit the usefulness of regression analyses for establishing high-risk registries.

Other pitfalls are posed by regression analysis. A high correlation coefficient between two variables does not mean that one causes the other. Danger exists in extrapolating or forecasting values of the independent variable lying beyond the sample range. Regression based on past data may not be a good predictor because of shifts in the disease patterns of the underlying population.

Neural Networks

Artificial intelligence and neural networks are a promising approach to segmenting the population on the basis of future cost from available historical data. Neural networks are a new statistical technique arising from the artificial-intelligence field (Russell and Norvig, 1998; Haykin, 1998). It has not yet achieved widespread recognition, understanding, and use.

The purpose of neural networks is to derive the best predictive model from available information. Their outputs are equations characterized by the r^2 of independent to outcome variables.

Neural networks can analyze many data fields virtually simultaneously, assert predictions toward the outcome of interest, determine the accuracy of their own predictions, and go on to generate even better models on the basis of their own analyses. They can also seek out patterns and examples from within large data sets, make numerical generalizations from them, and incorporate these associations into an overall predictive model. The rapid modeling and incremental improvements of neural networks are often described as a "learning" behavior simulating the functioning of the human mind.

Solving a problem using a neural network approach involves converting available information into numerical data. For predictive purposes, potentially useful patient information, such as age, demographics, blood glucose level, or blood creatinine level, is recognized for inclusion. Other information, like ICD9 inpatient discharge-diagnoses codes, is included as named rather than ordinal data. ICD9-coded diagnoses must be converted into the dichotomous presence or absence of a particular disease or clinical condition.

Once the data are put into a format recognizable to the neural network, the program "learns" by rearranging countless combinations and patterns among input variables to achieve a best fit according to the predictive value for the targeted outcome. An attractive feature is that the neural network constantly updates its model as new data are added. The result, for example, can be a "pattern of care" equation that best describes a managed care population segmented by future medical cost.

The methodology has enjoyed promising applications in both industry and health (Kemp, MacAulay, and Palcic, 1997; Hirshberg and Adar, 1997). A typical industry challenge is to maximize the yield of a chemical product. A variety of reaction attributes are known, such as the amount of each ingredient, reaction temperature, impurity levels, incubation time, pressure. The desired outputs are clear: yield and acceptable amount of impurities. Neural networks analyze results of a few experiments and predict an optimal set of input variables. Research and development in a chemical firm can use the neural network predictions to design more intelligent future experiments. New empirical data are incorporated into the network program for additional cycles of model improvement. The overall impact is to rapidly direct development of the most efficient production process, saving time and expense.

So far, clinical applications are scarce but promising. Pharmaceutical and device companies have found efficiencies by employing neural networks to develop predictive models from a clinical trial; they use the models to better direct the experimental approaches and to reduce the number of follow-up studies.

Segmenting a managed care population according to expected future medical cost is an essential capability for risk-bearing health organizations. Patterns of care can bypass limitations imposed by the assumptions of multiple regression modeling. Neural networks show promise of producing the best models because of their ability to deal with interrelated variables and nonlinear relationships.

Essential Characteristics of a High-Risk Population Segmentation Method

Essential accuracy characteristics are placed into a context by taking the *size of the population* into account. The *size of the high-risk registry* is important because this is the panel of patients on which proactive care management will be focused. Not only must the size be manageable from the standpoint of case management resources, but the *predictive value positive* must be high to substantiate an investment. *Sensitivity* must also be high in order to detect as many of the high-cost cases as possible. *Average $PMPM* after the high-risk patients appear on the registry can be accepted as a gross metric of how well the model is identifying high-cost cases.

A full set of these essential statistics must be established retrospectively, using multiple years of data. The first year data are used for application of predictive segmentation models. The second is the outcome year, where the ability of the model to predict cost outcomes is quantified.

Measuring Accuracy in Practice

All currently available predictive models are proprietary (see Table 14.1). Most organizations are not yet making direct comparisons of the accuracy of their offerings using epidemiological measures. To date consultants and health services researchers have not reported their predictive equations or results in any way that would permit direct comparisons.

Objective measures should be used to quantify the value of predictive segmentation models. Population size, registry size, sensitivity, and predictive value positive are the four measures with the most appealing clinically intuitive meaning. The fifth is the actual average $PMPM of those previously identified on the registry as high risk.

If a standard data set were available for a general population, like the data on Medicare claims furnished to health services researchers by HCFA, it could be used to analyze competing approaches. Because such a claims database is unavailable, to create a common testing ground each organization would have to supply data for two years, on which competing predictive models would be run. Because of variations among plans and groups in age profiles, prevalence of diseases, and regional practices, the results would be valid only for that one population.

In considering the results of such comparisons, organizations contemplating adopting one approach or another should consider nonquantitative factors as well. Chief among them are the differential prospects of constructively improving the care of high-risk patients. No list, no matter what its sensitivity and predictive value positive, will accomplish anything unless it can be used as the basis for carrying out constructive and measurable innovations in the care of the identified patients. Conversely, no change in their care will not produce results, even if there is perfect prior knowledge of who the Status One patients will be.

• • • • • • •

In this chapter epidemiological concepts were reviewed as a basis for gauging the accuracy of high-risk population predictive models. Commercially available computer programs for these purposes do not yet permit direct comparisons among them. A combination of population size, high-risk registry size, sensitivity, predictive value positive, and average $PMPM provides a necessary and sufficient view of the practical accuracy of such models. The same accuracy dimensions are equally applicable to high-risk population registries produced by empirical expert algorithms, multiple regression equations, or neural networks.

No matter how accurate the predictive capability of population segmenting methods, improvements in functional status and economic efficiency can come only from improving the processes and content of care for the highest-risk patients, regardless of the method of identification chosen.

15

· ·

Economics

Structural Aspects and Costs in Managed Health Care Populations

Much of managed care is an attempt to influence physicians to recommend the most cost-efficient and effective form of care. So far, HMO cost savings have been achieved primarily by discounting fees rather than by improving efficiencies and outcomes of clinical care.

To understand why this is the case and what to do about it, the reader must first understand structural aspects of HMOs and the health care delivery system. Armed with thorough knowledge of the current environment, clinical and administrative leaders can proceed with an effective medical management strategy for high-risk members. Making the care of Status One patients the first priority in a population health management strategy offers the greatest opportunity for economic efficiencies and clinical excellence in the near term; at the same time organizations can be preparing to expand the gains to the entire population as resources allow, one segment at a time.

Structural Aspects of Care Delivery

American health care providers from a variety of organizations are undergoing changing relationships with insurers and patients. From this alphabet soup of organizations emerges an alignment of clinical needs and economic incentives that can be exploited for the benefit of Status One patients (Weiner and de Lissovoy, 1993). This section provides a taxonomy of organizations and their essential characteristics.

Managed care arose in the United States as a means of providing clinical care to industrial employees and their families. This heritage of business payers remains strong in managed care through commercial HMO insurance plans offered to employers, business coalitions demanding low premiums on behalf of their workers, and the business-driven NCQA and its HEDIS quality measures.

Early in World War II the Kaiser Steel Corporation could not ensure adequate health care for workers. It was importing entire families from around the country into burgeoning communities surrounding its West Coast shipyards. Expanding on a prepaid health care model for Los Angeles civil-service workers and contemporary English models, Kaiser built its own medical facilities and hired physicians and nurses. Employees prepaid part of their health care premiums by payroll deduction, and the employer paid the larger share. Complete health services were provided within Kaiser's own network of employed physicians, clinics, and hospitals. The circumstances of war and scarcity of clinicians remaining after the draft combined to stifle objections from the American Medical Association, which labeled this type of prepaid care a threat to physician autonomy and FFS medicine. Kaiser Steel also benefited in other ways. The cost of building clinics and hospitals was included as part of cost-plus military contracts for steel and warships. The clinical staff it hired were exempt from the draft as essential war workers.

Kaiser Permanente, spun off as a charitable foundation after the war, became a not-for-profit HMO. It combines insurance functions by offering health plans through employers and direct medical care. In industry jargon, it is a staff-model HMO, one that owns its "bricks and mortar" clinics and hospitals and employs salaried clinical providers.

Today, a variety of health care organizations exist, although few still have a convergence of actuarial risk and links to health care delivery. In the Kaiser Permanente staff model, insurance and clinical functions are in the same organization. Many people still believe that the unity of insurance and health care delivery characterizes the HMO. But as insurers have increasingly divested their clinics and health care delivery systems to increase efficiencies, it is currently rare to have the two functions within the same entity.

It is appropriate to review and become conversant with the variety of MCOs in order to appreciate the opportunity posed by population health management. MCOs that retain financial risk and are constructively engaged with clinical care have both the incentive and the means to influence the quality and costs of health care.

MCOs are legally licensed corporate entities, organized and operated as health insurers within the states in which they do business. They are authorized to sell insurance to employers, segmented into small-, medium-, and large-group product lines, and to individuals. Each insurance offering is characterized by a defined set of covered health benefits regulated by the insurance laws in each state.

For-Profit and Not-for-Profit Structures

MCO corporate entities can be either nonprofit or for-profit entities. Not-for-profits are maintained as charitable community organizations. Excess revenues over expenses are not taxed as profits but may be held as reserves. Nonprofit MCOs tend to have a longer-term focus than their for-profit cousins. Accountability, however, is somewhat diffuse, with large boards of directors representing a variety of community interests. In New England, for example, nonprofit MCOs dominate the managed-care landscape, with Tufts Health Plan, Harvard-Pilgrim Health Care, Blue Cross/Blue Shield, and Fallon Community Health Plan recognizable names both regionally and nationally. Kaiser remains a dominant presence on the West Coast and has operations in several other states.

For-profit MCOs are owned by their shareholders. Their profits are taxable as business income, as in any corporation. They tend to have a shorter-term focus on the latest quarterly earnings per share and revenue growth. The goal is clear and specific: to maximize shareholder value. Examples include major corporations whose shares are traded on the major stock exchanges—Aetna/U.S. Health Care, United Healthcare, Pacificare Health Systems, and CIGNA.

Regulation

Both for-profit and not-for profit MCOs are regulated by state divisions of insurance to ensure required levels of dollar reserves and some insurance rates—for example, rates for Blue Cross/Blue Shield supplemental Medicare insurance. Self-insured businesses involved in interstate commerce are exempt from state regulations. ERISA, a 1975 law originally intended to protect private sector retirement accounts, also gives such companies broad discretion in health benefits coverage for their employees.

Levels of Benefits and Clinician Choice

Managed care organizations can be further classified based on the products they offer in the marketplace; these products include HMOs, preferred provider plans (PPOs), point-of-service plans (POSs), and provider-sponsored networks (PSNs). Although all these insurance products are loosely referred to as "managed care," they differ in the extent of clinician choice and medical management. *Medical management* refers to the set of policies, procedures, and practices designed to provide the most appropriate and cost-efficient care for members of an MCO. HMOs are the most limiting of the MCOs, restricting care to providers within the HMO network who abide by its utilization rules and clinical guidelines. HMOs have different provider arrangements. Some own their clinics and employ clinicians, as does the original Kaiser Permanente model; they may have an exclusive medical group as do Mayo, Cleveland, Ochsner, and Marshfield clinics; or they may be a group of independent community practices and clinicians contractually linked as an IPA.

PPOs have a larger provider network and fewer utilization controls than HMOs. POS plans differ little from traditional indemnity FFS care except that physician providers are paid on a discounted fee schedule.

For commercial managed care, the employer defines the level of insurance risk. Employers may purchase a fully insured premium for their employees' health care. Alternatively they may be self-insured and utilize the HMO for its provider network and to administer its employees' health claims (administrative services only or as third party administrator). Many employers have mixed levels of risk— for example, they may carve out pharmaceuticals, infertility treatments, mental health, or chiropractic services, while retaining actuarial risk on the rest of their employees' medical care.

Typical Benefit Plans

Benefits vary according to plan type (see Table 15.1). Premiums are progressively higher among HMOs, PPOs, and POS plans, reflecting higher costs associated with each.

HMO benefit coverage is restricted to network providers for covered services. Patients going out of the network will typically pay out of pocket, unless an emergency has occurred and the HMO agrees to pay for it. Prior PCP authorization is required for specialists and costly diagnostic services. Prescription drugs are usually covered by commercial HMO plans, although most have a predefined formulary of authorized pharmaceuticals and a restricted network of pharmacies.

A PPO has fewer restrictions on the provider network and benefits. Members may see physicians out of the network if they accept higher copayments and deductibles. A PCP may not be required to preauthorize hospitalization, specialty care, and diagnostic services.

The POS plans are the least restrictive. POS is most like FFS medicine; the chief difference is that a POS provider is paid from a

Table 15.1. Typical Benefit Plans

Plan	Covered Services	Noncovered Services
HMO	All ambulatory and physician office care	Alternative therapies
		Nonemergency out-of-area care
	Inpatient	Nonauthorized care
	Emergency room	Out-of-network providers
	Ancillary rehabilitation	
	Skilled nursing facility	
	Prescriptions	
	Preventive dental services	
	Mental health and substance abuse services	
	Out-of-area emergencies	
PPO	Same as HMO, with deductibles or co-insurance for out-of-network services	Same as HMO, except plan may not have a PCP and not require referrals
POS	Same as PPO, with deductibles but no network distinctions	Same as PPO, often does not include prescriptions

standard fee schedule. There are usually no preferred network providers.

Provider-sponsored networks (PSNs) are risk-bearing provider groups. New to the health care landscape, PSNs are growing as insurers; they increasingly assign risk to their contracted provider organizations. Medicare is starting to allow PSNs to sponsor Medicare managed care plans. PSN networking and clinical practices are likely to be similar to group-model HMOs; they are characterized by strong policies requiring patients to seek their care from providers and ancillary services within the network. Like an insurer, the PSN will most often retain risk for clinical care it does not provide directly—for example, hospital care, skilled nursing facilities, and dispensing pharmacies.

A risk contracting organization (RCO) is any managed care delivery organization (physician hospital organization or PHO, IDS,

IPA) that contracts with managed care plans and accepts financial risk for a population for a defined scope of clinical services. As an organization of clinical providers, it is able to align financial and quality incentives. RCOs administer medical care and the distribution of compensation to physicians and other providers. Typically they cover themselves for unanticipated catastrophic cases by purchasing stop-loss insurance. RCOs may be either for-profit or not-for profit corporate entities.

RCOs include medical groups (physician corporations), PHOs, and physician practice management (PPM) companies. Many readers will be familiar with consolidations of urban teaching hospitals in New York, San Francisco, Boston, Philadelphia, St. Louis, and a number of other cities into PHOs that use their enlarged bargaining power to negotiate capitation arrangements and per diem rates with insurers.

PPMs grew dramatically as they raised capital in the financial markets, acquired physician practices, and, in turn, negotiated global medical risk contracts with insurers. PhyCor and MedPartners are among such organizations; they are as visible to clinicians and insurers as they are to readers of the *Wall Street Journal*. More recently they have fallen from favor in the investment community as administrative efficiencies they had hoped to achieve could not be parlayed into profitable operations. By 1999 MedPartners was actively divesting itself from its recently acquired medical practices in favor of its pharmaceutical benefits division.

RCOs seek to obtain medical management responsibilities from insurers in a process dubbed "delegation" by the NCQA. They also acquire computer systems and technology to manage administration and billing for the care they provide. Their major strategies are aimed at improving the coordination and functional status of their most acute and chronically ill patients, restricting referral patterns to within the RCO, and achieving shared quality goals and financial incentives.

Successful medical and administrative leadership in RCOs works to achieve among member clinicians a sense of partnership, shared vision, accountability for key measures, customer orientation, and a focus on improving and managing care. High-risk population health management holds appeal for RCOs because of its sharp focus on few members, near-term financial outcomes, and resonance with altruistic clinical motivations.

The reader may note that the functions of the globally capitated RCOs are virtually identical to those of the original staff-model HMOs, which retained financial risk and delivered services. Growth of the RCO model while the old staff models languish can be linked to consumer demand for provider choice, the geographical convenience that staff models cannot offer, and cost efficiencies that salaried physicians have generally not achieved.

Costs of Health Care Delivery

Many factors are driving the inflation of health care costs in the United States.

Demographic Shifts

The population is aging as the post-World War II baby boomers progress into middle age. Relative to their numbers, senior citizens consume many more health care services as measured in dollars than their working-age counterparts. The leading cohort of boomers will reach age sixty-five in 2010. At that timer fewer younger people will be in the workforce and contributing to social welfare programs, Medicare, and Social Security. The long-term viability of these programs has already emerged as an important political issue. Year by year the average age of the population increases, with a commensurate upward drift in the demand for health services.

Reimbursements

The FFS reimbursement system, which was the national norm until the growth of capitated, prepaid managed care, has an inherent bias toward more care. Patients rely heavily on the therapeutic recom-mendations of their providers. As long as clinicians are paid more for any additional care, they have an incentive to give more and more complex care. FFS remains common. Even the areas of the country with the highest market penetration of managed care do not approach 100 percent membership in MCOs. Los Angeles County, for example, a Southern California area generally assumed to be dominated by managed care, has some 60 percent of eligible people in PPO-type plans.

PPO fee schedules retain FFS incentives at the provider level. Such fee structures encourage providers to recommend high uti-lization surgery and other invasive procedures. Similar perverse incentives exist in favor of more care, while lower reimbursements encourage the provider to "churn" ambulatory patient volume.

Hospital Overcapacity

The Hill-Burton Act was a piece of federal legislation that subsi-dized community-hospital construction. Medicare reimburses hos-pitals for both the direct costs of care and the depreciation of buildings. FFS frequently incented more care of the inpatient vari-ety. The result was a sustained building of hospital-bed capacity that came to far outstrip the need.

As MCOs became the distributors of health care funding, hos-pitals faced a transition from being revenue generators to being cost centers. The tendency to fill unused hospital beds instead of using less costly community alternatives, when appropriate, remains a driver of health care cost inflation.

Physician Oversupply

By many measures the United States has too many physicians, espe-cially in certain clinical specialties. In the FFS environment, physi-cian providers could modulate the demand and reimbursements for their services. The more physicians, the more demand for health care services.

New Pharmaceuticals

The most profitable portion of the health care sector is pharmaceutical companies. Like innovations in all industries, new drug discoveries are afforded patent protection for seventeen years. A breakthrough drug enjoys immediate demand from specialists, some of whom may have achieved academic recognition by leading the new drug's clinical trials. Until a rival obtains Food and Drug Administration approval to market another agent in the same class, the drug company effectively has a monopoly, which allows it to recover its development costs and make a profit.

Diagnostic, Therapeutic, and Device Innovations

Innovations are not confined to new drugs. New and costly approaches to clinical care abound. Entire classes of care did not exist within our memories. Diagnostic computerized axial tomography, magnetic resonance imaging, major organ transplants, cardiac bypass surgery, and test-tube babies are but a few innovations now taken as routine that did not exist when the majority of clinicians were in training. The tendency is to use the new technologies aggressively once they are available, especially in the FFS environment.

Expanded Services

Many states have mandated services that could be construed as elective or unnecessary. For example, legislation has mandated two-day hospital stays for uncomplicated labor and delivery in many locales and insurance coverage of unlimited attempts at in vitro fertilization.

Patient Expectations

Many patients expect the most specialized physician and most advanced techniques for their ailments. For years under FFS arrangements, patients could see the cardiologist for high blood pressure and the endocrinologist for uncomplicated diabetes mellitus. The most aggressive diagnostic tests were available for the asking. If one physician thought they might not be appropriate, one could shop around for a physician who did.

A cultural change that leads most patients to desire the most appropriate care for their condition, preferring a generalist with whom they have a long-term relationship unless the challenge is particularly complex, may take many years of managed care to bring about. The legacy of FFS medicine, no personal accountability for costs, and an environment awash in specialists leads to the common patient expectation for specialty and high-technology care, regardless of intrinsic clinical need.

Defensive Medicine

Litigation has become an all too frequent recourse in American society. Some clinicians perform diagnostic evaluations and care, in part, as a defense against potential lawsuits. The high frequency of Cesarean sections with the routine use of fetal monitors is an example. Obstetricians faced with an equivocal fetal-monitor reading would often rather perform the surgical birthing procedure than face a ruinous malpractice suit in the unlikely event of a birth injury.

Physician Education and Specialization

Medical education and reimbursement has for years favored specialization. Specialists tend to practice a more resource-intensive brand of medicine when compared with generalists treating the same kinds of conditions. Like the fabled hammer, which views the world as so many nails, the surgical and medical specialists have been molded to view clinical situations as opportunities for them to apply their latest surgical or invasive diagnostic techniques.

International Comparisons

The provision of health services in other developed countries furnishes a diversity of models far different from ours. Common threads suggest opportunities for cost and quality controls rarely seized in the United States. Population health management exploits several characteristics common to generally successful foreign health care systems.

Among single-insured managed care populations in the United States, all four common attributes of internationally successful cost controls exist:

Unity of the finance and delivery of health care in one organization

Fixed global budgets for all care

Adequate minimum benefits package

Universal access

These attributes are found in delivery systems globally capped by insurers, HMOs retaining risk, and PSNs. Provider organizations retaining actuarial risk are in the best position to modulate care toward cost-effective alternatives while remaining immediately responsible for clinical quality. HMO insurers are more distant from the delivery of care but share the motivation. Other producers of health care goods and services have a stake in outcomes but are variously removed from the front lines of health care or from the immediate consequences of expending resources on such care.

. . . .

In this chapter the diverse MCO network and benefit schemes as well as current medical management practices have been examined. Although the pressures fueling health care cost inflation are many, international comparisons demonstrate that it is possible to spend less on health care, to have a generally satisfied populace, and to improve measures of population health. High-risk population health management can be an attractive medical management strategy for risk-bearing provider groups because of its sharp focus on relatively few people, as well as their large impact on costs. An RCO can directly influence the way that care is rendered for Status One patients. Insurers are a step removed from managing the delivery of care, but their financial incentives are similar to those of the risk-bearing RCO.

Part V

. . . .

Putting It Together

16

Summary
Best Practices in High-Risk Population Management

M anaged care organizations aspiring to master the current cost-constrained environment and to position themselves for a more quality-driven future should seriously consider adopting the high-risk population health management strategy. Segmenting a population by predictive clinical registries, focusing first on Status One patients, modulating clinical service intensity according to the likelihood of incurring future costs, and producing metrics meaningful to the managed care leadership will be among the hallmarks of successful organizations.

Other types of medical management strategies fit into the overall picture according to their expected contributions to care of the highest-risk patient groups. All clinical programs should be held accountable for results, using the same kind of business and clinical metrics applied elsewhere in managed care. This chapter outlines key components of high-risk population management.

Once the care for high-risk Status One patients is optimal, other direct medical management approaches can be adopted incrementally to address the needs of other population segments according to need and economic opportunity. When health plans compete on the basis of clinical quality, as anticipated, plans and groups that have achieved quantifiable results with high-risk population health management and are making progress with major disease initiatives will be in an excellent competitive position. In the meantime, population health management, affording first priority to Status One members, will serve plans, group practices, and their patients well during the cost-driven present.

Segment the Population

Clinical leaders segment the population from already available databases, identifying patients by risk group and disease and formulating patient registries. Collecting input information from existing electronically accessible claims, pharmacy, and laboratory data is a strategy possessing favorable trade-offs among cost, timeliness, and clinical usefulness. The first step of population health management is to pursue the segmentation strategy that produces clinically actionable registries. High-risk patient registries are updated frequently in order to accommodate these unstable, comorbid, socially complex patients.

Focus on Status One Patients First

The next step is to winnow medical management strategies down to those addressing Status One patient needs. Medical management program design focuses first and most intensely on Status One patients. Content and efficiency of care should be optimal for these highest-risk members before an organization embarks on programs farther along the "pathway to clinical excellence."

Assess and Manage the Care of Each High-Risk Patient

We recommend care managers use a psychosocial model of care to supplement the usual clinical activities. Care planning should incorporate the tenets of mass customization rather than of guideline-oriented, single-disease programs. Innovations by clinicians, nurses, and support personnel should be encouraged.

Conduct Research in Parallel

Many aspects of population-based care for high-risk patients will benefit from research. The relative efficacy of various interventions remains unquantified, although overall economic results are compelling. The challenge to the leadership of managed care organizations is to focus the organization on the care of Status One patients now while supporting research when the opportunity arises. Conversely, delaying aggressive programs because the medical and scientific base is incomplete causes an organization to miss a major opportunity to serve a needy patient group and positively affect the financial bottom line.

Create Synergy

All types of clinical programs providing the unstable and costly patient with better and more cost-efficient care should be closely aligned with Status One patient care. In particular, hospitalist programs that aim to shorten the length of costly inpatient stays complement proactive Status One patient care, which can be characterized as an admission-avoidance strategy. Similarly, disease management programs concentrating on the few and the most needy complement the high-risk population management strategy.

Use Technology to Advantage

Computerized aids to population segmentation and care planning should be enlisted in the effort. Creative intranet applications can fulfill the longstanding need to link patchwork systems of care on behalf of the small set of the most needy. Essential information can be shared across the continuum of care for the small set of highest-risk patients without the need for a fully automated medical record or a large investment in computer and communications technology.

Employ Meaningful Metrics

Leaders should assess clinical management efforts on behalf of Status One patients and disease initiatives with the same type of metrics used to lead managed care organizations—namely, measures of near-term cost and resource efficiency.

• • • • • •

At the present time systematic improvements in Status One patient care are virtually unknown within managed care organizations. Recognition of this small group of needy patients, their unique needs, and opportunities to improve their care is minimal.

High-risk population health management, starting with Status One patients, poses a rare opportunity to concentrate medical management strategies, an approach that arises out of a convergence of medical necessity and financial imperatives. It is up to managed care leaders to recognize the opportunity and to creatively serve these most needy and unstable members.

References

Alderfer, C. P. "An Empirical Test of a New Theory of Human Needs." *Organizational Behavior and Human Performance,* 1969, *4,* 141–175.

American Medical Association. *Directory of Practice Parameters.* Chicago: American Medical Association, 1998.

Anderson, G., and Steinberg, E. "Predicting Hospital Readmissions in the Medicare Population." *Inquiry,* 1995, *22,* 251–258.

Barsky, A. J. *The Worried Sick: Our Troubled Quest for Wellness.* Boston: Little, Brown, 1988.

Beck, A., and others. "A Randomized Trial of Group Outpatient Visits for Chronically Ill Older HMO Members: Thew Cooperative Health Care Clinic." *Journal of the American Geriatric Society,* 1997, *45*(5), 543–549.

Berkman, B., Miller, S., Holmes, W., and Boander, E. "Predicting Elderly Cardiac Patients at Risk for Readmission." *Social Work Health Care,* 1991, *16,* 21–38.

Berkman, B., Walker, S., Boander, E., and Holmes, W. "Early Unplanned Readmissions to Social Work of Elderly Patients: Factors Predicting Who Needs Follow-Up Services." *Social Work Health Care,* 1991, *17,* 103–119.

Berman, S. (ed.). "Making Good on the Promise: Disseminating and Implementing Practice Guidelines." *Quality Review Bulletin,* 1992, *18*(12), 393–482.

Berwick, D. M., Godfrey, A. B., and Roessner, J. *Curing Health Care: New Strategies for Quality Improvement.* San Francisco: Jossey-Bass, 1990.

Bishop, J. F., and Macarounas-Kirchman, K. "The Pharmacoeconomics of Cancer Therapies." *Seminars in Oncology,* 1997, *24,* S19–106–S19–111.

Blumenthal, D., and Buntin, M. B. "Carve Outs: Definitions, Experience, and Choice Among Candidate Conditions." *American Journal of Managed Care,* 1998, *4,* SP45–SP57.

Bodenheimer, T. "The HMO Backlash—Righteous or Reactionary?" *New England Journal of Medicine*, 1996, *335*(21), 1601–1604.

Boult C., Pacala, J. T., and Boult, L. B. "Targeting Elders for Geriatric Evaluation and Management: Reliability, Validity and Practicality of a Questionnaire." *Aging Clinical and Experimental Research*, 1995, *7*, 159–164.

Boult, C., and others. "Screening Elders for Risk of Hospital Readmission." *Journal of the American Geriatric Society*, 1993, *41*, 811–817.

Bowling, A. *Measuring Disease—A Review of Disease-Specific Quality of Life Measurement Scales*. Bristol, Pa.: Open University Press, 1995.

Burns, F. J., Seddon, P., Saul, M., and Zeidel, M. L. "The Cost of Caring for End-Stage Kidney Disease Patients: An Analysis Based on Hospital Financial Transaction Records." *Journal of the American Society of Nephrology*, 1998, *9*(5), 884–890.

Burns, R., and Nichols, L. O. "Factors Predicting Readmission of Older General Medicine Patients." *Journal of General Internal Medicine*, 1991, *5*, 389–393.

Cardinale, V. (ed.). *Drug Topics Red Book*. Montvale, N.J.: Medical Economics Company, 1998.

Clark, D. O., and others. "A Chronic Disease Score with Empirically Derived Weights." *Medical Care*, 1995, *33*(8), 783–795.

Codman, E. A. "The Product of a Hospital." *Surgery, Gynecology, Obstetrics*, 1914, *18*, 491–496.

Codman, E. A. *A Study in Hospital Efficiency: As Demonstrated by the Care Report of the First Five Years of a Private Hospital*. Boston: Thomas Todd, 1916.

Coleman, E. A., and others. "Predicting Hospitalization and Functional Status in Older Health Plan Enrollees: Are Administrative Data as Accurate as Self-Report?" *Journal of the American Geriatric Society*, 1998, *46*(4), 35 419–425.

Computers, Science and Telecommunications Board, Commission on Physical Sciences. *For the Record: Protecting Electronic Health Information*. Washington, D.C.: National Academy Press, 1997.

Corrigan, J. M., and Martin, J. B. "Identification of Factors Associated with Hospital Readmission and Development of a Predictive Model." *Health Services Research*, 1992, *27*, 81–101.

Covey, S. R. *The Seven Basic Habits of Highly Effective People*. New York: Simon & Schuster, 1989.

Crane, J., and others. "Markers of Risk of Asthma Death or Readmission in the 12 Months Following a Hospital Admission for Asthma." *International Journal of Epidemiology*, 1992, *21*, 737–744.

Davidson, G. "Does Inappropriate Use Explain Small-Area Variations in the Use of Health Care Services?" *Health Services Research*, 1993, *28*, 389–400.

Delbanco, T. L. "Enriching the Doctor-Patient Relationship by Inviting the Patient's Perspective." *Annals of Internal Medicine*, 1992, *116*(5), 414–417.

Deming, W. E. *Out of the Crisis*. Cambridge, Mass.: MIT Press, 1986.

Diabetes Control and Complications Trial Research Group. "The Effect of Intensive Treatment of Diabetes on the Development and Progression of Long-Term Complications in Insulin-Dependent Diabetes Mellitus." *New England Journal of Medicine*, 1993, *329*, 977–986.

Diabetes Control and Complications Trial Research Group. "Lifetime Benefits and Costs of Intensive Therapy as Practiced in the Diabetes Control and Complications Trial." *Journal of the American Medical Association*, 1996, *276*, 1409–1415.

Diabetes Control and Complications Trial Study Group. "Resource Utilization and Costs of Care in the Diabetes Control and Complications Trial." *Diabetes Care*, 1995, *18*, 1468–1478.

Diabetes Control and Complications Trial Study Group, Testa, M. A., and Simonson, D. C. "Health Economics Benefits and Quality of Life During Improved Glycemic Control in Patients with Type 2 Diabetes Mellitus." *Journal of the American Medical Association*, 1998, *280*(17), 1490–1496.

Donabedian, A. "Evaluating the Quality of Medical Care." *Milbank Memorial Fund Quarterly*, 1966, *44*(3), pt. 2, 166–203.

Eisenberg, J. M. *Doctors' Decisions and Cost of Medical Care*. Ann Arbor, Mich.: Health Administration Press, 1986.

Ellis, R. P., and Ash, A. "Refinements to the Diagnostic Cost Group (DCG) Model." *Inquiry*, Winter 1995/1996, *32*, 418–429.

Ellrodt, G., and others. "Evidence-Based Disease Management." *Journal of the American Medical Association*, 1997, *278*(20), 1687–1692.

Epstein, R. S., and Sherwood, L. M. "From Outcomes Research to Disease Management: A Guide for the Perplexed." *Annals of Internal Medicine*, 1996, *124*, 832–837.

Eraker, S. "Understanding and Improving Patient Compliance." *Annals of Internal Medicine*, 1984, *100*(2), 258–268.

Fehtke, C. C., Smith, I., and Johnson, N. "Risk Factors Affecting Readmission of the Elderly into the Health Care System." *Medical Care*, 1986, *24*, 429–437.

Fetter, R. B. (ed.). "DRGs—Their Design and Development." Ann Arbor, Mich.: Health Administration Press, 1991.

Field, M. J., and Lohr, K. N. *Guidelines for Clinical Practice: From Development to Use.* Washington, D.C.: National Academy Press, 1992.

Forman, S. A., Kelliher, M., and Wood, G. "Clinical Improvement with Bottom-Line Impact: Custom Care Planning for Patients with Acute and Chronic Illnesses in a Managed Care Setting." *American Journal of Managed Care*, 1997, 3(7), 1039–1048.

Frasure-Smith, N., and others. "Depression Following Myocardial Infarction." *Journal of the American Medical Association*, 1993, 270, 1819–1825.

Goonan, K. J. *The Juran Prescription: Clinical Quality Management.* San Francisco: Jossey-Bass, 1995.

Greene, J. "Plans Bowing Out of Report Card Projects." *American Medical News*, Nov. 2, 1998a.

Greene, J. "Sizing Up the Sickest: Clues About Patients in Danger of a Costly Medical Crisis Are Already Sitting in Your Database." *Hospitals & Health Networks*, 1998b, 72(9), 28.

Hagland, M. "Web-Based Medical Information Systems Used by Three Medical Centers." *Health Management Technology*, 1998, 19(4), 22.

Hanna, D. P. *Designing Organizations for High Performance.* Reading, Mass.: Addison-Wesley, 1988.

Harris, J. M. "Disease Management: New Wine in New Bottles?" *Annals of Internal Medicine*, 1996, 124, 838–842.

Haykin, S. S. *Neural Networks: A Comprehensive Foundation.* Upper Saddle River, N.J.: Prentice-Hall, 1998.

Hirshberg, A., and Adar, R. "Artificial Neural Networks in Medicine." *Israel Journal of Medical Sciences*, 1997, 33(10), 700–702.

Hoffman, C., Rice, D., Sung, H.Y. "Persons With Chronic Conditions. Their Prevalence and Costs." *Journal of the American Medical Association*, 1996, 276(18), 1473–1479.

Holdford, D. A. "Barriers to Disease Management." *American Journal of Health System Pharmacy*, 1996, 53, 2093–2096.

International Classification of Diseases: Clinical Modification. (5th ed.) Clinical Modification. Los Angeles: Practice Management Improvement Corporation, 1998.

Ishikawa, K. *What Is Total Quality Control?* Upper Saddle River, N.J.: Prentice-Hall, 1985.

Juran, J. M. *Juran on Planning for Quality.* New York: Free Press, 1988.

Juran, J. M. *Juran on Quality by Design.* New York: Free Press, 1992.

Kassirer, J. "The Quality of Care and the Quality of Measuring It." *New England Journal of Medicine*, 1993a, 329, 1263–1265.

Kassirer, J. "The Use and Abuse of Practice Profiles." *New England Journal of Medicine*, 1993b, *330*(9), 634–635.

Kemp, R. A., MacAulay, C., and Palcic, B. "Opening the Black Box: The Relationship Between Neural Networks and Linear Discriminant Functions." *Annals of Cellular Pathology*, 1997, *14*(1), 19–30.

Kirchner, C. G., and others. *Physicians' Current Procedural Terminology*. Chicago: American Medical Association, 1996.

Kleinbaum, D. G. (ed.). *Applied Regression Analysis and Other Multivariable Methods*. (3rd ed.) Duxbury Press, 1997.

Kleinbaum, D. G., Kupper, L. L., and Morgenstern, H. *Epidemiologic Research: Principles and Quantitative Methods*. New York: Wiley, 1982.

Kongstvedt, P. R. *The Managed Health Care Handbook*. (2nd ed.) Gaithersburg, Md.: Aspen, 1993.

Kuhn, T. S. *The Structure of Scientific Revolutions*. (3rd ed.) Chicago: University of Chicago Press, 1996.

Kurowski, B. "Cancer Carve Outs, Specialty Networks, and Disease Management: A Review of Their Evolution, Effectiveness, and Prognosis." *American Journal of Managed Care*, 1998, *4*, SP71–SP89.

Larkin, H. "Not All Health Plans Live Up to Potential." *American Medical News*, 1997, *40*(39), 1, 30.

Last, J. M., and Wallace, R. B. (eds.). *Maxey-Rosenau-Last Public Health & Preventive Medicine*. (13th ed.) East Norwalk, Conn.: Appleton & Lang, 1992.

Leveille, S. G., and others. "Preventing Disability and Managing Chronic Illness in Frail Older Adults: A Randomized Trial of a Community-Based Partnership with Primary Care." *Journal of the American Geriatric Society*, 1998, *46*, 1–9.

Lorig, K., and others. *Living a Healthy Life with Chronic Conditions*. Palo Alto, Calif.: Bull Publishing, 1994.

Maslow, A. H. "A Theory of Human Motivation." *Psychology Review*, July 1943, 370–396.

Mazze, R., Strock, E., Etzweiller, D., and Simonson, G. *Staged Diabetes Management™ Complications Manual*. Minneapolis: International Diabetes Center, Institute for Research and Education, HealthSystem Minnesota, 1997.

Melanka, D. J., and O'Connor, G. T. "A Regional Collaborative Effort for CQI in Cardiovascular Disease—Northern New England Cardiovascular Study Group." *Joint Commission Journal on Quality Improvement*, 1995, *21*(11), 627–633.

Melanka, D. J., and O'Connor, G. T. "The Northern New England Cardiovascular Disease Study Group: A Regional Collaborative Effort for Continuous

Quality Improvement in Cardiovascular Disease." *Joint Commission Journal on Quality Improvement*, 1998, 24(10), 594–600.

Miller, W. R., and Rolnick, S. *Motivational Interviewing—Preparing People to Change Addictive Behavior*. New York: Guilford Press, 1991.

Morris, P., and others. "Association of Depression with 10-Year Poststroke Mortality." *American Journal of Psychiatry*, 1993, 150, 124–129.

Mossey, J. M., and others. "The Effects of Persistent Depressive Symptoms on Hip Fracture Recovery." *Journal of Gerontology*, 1990, 45(5), 163–168.

National Committee on Quality Assurance. *Standards for Managed Care Accreditation*. Washington, D.C.: National Committee on Quality Assurance, 1998.

Noble, J. (ed.). *Textbook of Primary Care Medicine*. (2nd ed.) St. Louis, Mo.: Mosby-Year Book, 1997.

Oleson, J. D. *Pathways to Agility: Mass Customization in Action*. New York: Wiley, 1998.

Pacala, J. T., Boult, C., and Boult, L. B. "Predictive Validity of a Questionnaire That Identifies Elders at Risk for Hospital Admission." *Journal of the American Geriatric Society*, 1995, 43, 374–377.

Pacala, J. T., Boult, C., Reed, R. L., and Aliberti, E. "Predictive Validity of the P_{ra} Instrument Among Older Recipients of Managed Care." *Journal of the American Geriatric Society*, 1997, 45(5), 614–617.

Pezella, S. M., O'Mara, P., and Donahue, J. N. "An Ambulatory Care Program for Managing High-Risk Congestive Heart Failure Patients." *Journal of Clinical Outcomes Management*, 1997, 4(3), 27–35.

Prager, L. O. "NCQA Delays Grading on Outcomes." *American Medical News*, Aug. 17, 1998.

Prochaska, J. O., Norcross, J. C., and DiClemente, C. C. *Changing for Good*. New York: Avon, 1994.

Quick, R. "In the Middle: Case Managers Want to Give Patients the Best Care, but Must Also Control Costs. It's a Constant Struggle." *Wall Street Journal*, Oct. 23, 1997, pp. 18, 20.

Rich, M. W., and Beckman, V. "Early Readmission of Elderly Patients with Congestive Heart Failure." *American Journal of Geriatric Cardiology*, 1996, 5(3), 32–36.

Rich, M. W., and Freedland, K. E. "Effects of DRGs on Three Month Readmission Rate of Geriatric Patients with Congestive Heart Failure." *American Journal of Public Health*, 1988, 8, 680–682.

Rich, M. W., and others. "Prevention of Readmission in Elderly Patients with Congestive Heart Failure: Results of a Prospective, Randomized Pilot Study." *Journal of General Internal Medicine*, 1993, 8, 585–590.

Rich, M. W., and others. "A Multidisciplinary Intervention to Prevent the Readmission of Elderly Patients with Congestive Heart Failure." *New England Journal of Medicine*, 1995, *333*, 1190–1195.

Rothman, K. J. (ed.). Modern Epidemiology. (2nd ed.). Philadelphia: Lippincott, 1998.

Russell, S. J., and Norvig, P. *Artificial Intelligence: A Modern Approach.* Upper Saddle River, N.J.: Prentice-Hall, 1998.

Schore, J., Brown, R., Cheh, V., and Schneider, B. *Costs and Consequences of Case Management for Medicare Beneficiaries.* Princeton, N.J.: Mathematica Policy Research, 1997.

Scott, L. "Disease Management Faces Obstacles." *Modern Healthcare*, June 12, 1995.

Skolnick, J. A. "NCQA: Quality Through Evaluation." *Journal of the American Medical Association*, 1997, *278*(19), 1555–1562.

Smeltzer, S. C., Suddarth, D. S., and Bare, B. (eds.). *Brunner and Suddarth's Textbook of Medical-Surgical Nursing.* (8th ed.) Philadelphia: Lippincott, 1996.

Snyder, C. R. *The Psychology of Hope.* New York: Free Press, 1994.

Steen, E. S. (ed.). *The Computer-Based Patient Record: An Essential Technology for Health Care.* Washington, D.C.: National Academy Press, 1998.

Stewart, A. L., and others. "Functional Status and Well-Being of Patients with Chronic Conditions: Results from the Medical Outcomes Study." *Journal of the American Medical Association*, 1989, *262*, 907–913.

Testa, M. A., and Simonson, D. C. "Health Economic Benefits and Quality of Life During Improved Glycemic Control in Patients with Type 2 Diabetes Mellitus, a Randomized, Controlled, Double-Blind Trial." *Journal of the American Medical Association*, 1998, *280*(17), 1490–1496.

Thorn, K. "The Birth of Third Generation Case Management." *Journal of Case Management*, 1993, *4*, 12–16.

Vibbert, S., Migdail, K. J., Strickland, D., and Youngs, M. T. *The Medical Outcomes and Guideline Sourcebook.* New York: Faulkner & Gray, 1994.

Vinson, J. M., and others. "Early Readmission of Elderly Patients with Congestive Heart Failure." *Journal of the American Geriatric Society*, 1990, 38, 1290–1295.

Wahba, M. A., and Bridwell, L. G. "Maslow Reconsidered: A Review of the Research on the Need Hierarchy Theory." *Organizational Behavior and Human Performance*, 1976, *15*, 212–240.

Wanous, J. P., and Zwany, A. "A Cross-Sectional Test of Need Hierarchy Theory." *Organizational Behavior and Human Performance*, 1977, *18*, 78–97.

Ware, J. E., Snow, K. K., Kosinski, M., and Gandek, B. *SF-36 Health Survey, Manual and Interpretation Guide*. Boston: Health Institute, New England Medical Center, 1995.

Weiner, J. P., and de Lissovoy, G. "Razing a Tower of Babel: A Taxonomy for Managed Care and Health Insurance Plans." *Journal of Health Politics, Policy and Law*, 1993, *18*(1), 75–103.

Weingarten, S., and Ellrodt, A. G. "The Case for Intensive Dissemination: Adoption of Practice Guidelines in Coronary Care Units." *Quality Review Bulletin*, 1992, *18*(12), 449–455.

Wennberg, J. E., Freeman, J. L., and Culp, W. J. "Are Hospital Services Rationed in New Haven or Over-utilized in Boston?" *Lancet*, 1987, *1*, 1185–1189.

Exhibits

• •

Exhibit A. Sample Letter of Introduction from the Primary-Care Physician.

March 11, 2001

Mr. Keith Forest
9 Inchon Way
Anytown, MA 01899

Dear Mr. Forest,

Your health and well being are important to me as your primary-care physician and to the health care team at the ABC Medical Group. To help us best understand your health concerns, please complete the attached questionnaire and return it in the enclosed self-addressed envelope. This questionnaire is confidential and will assist us in planning your care.

I have asked Ann Frost, your care manager who works closely with me, to contact you at home. Ann will coordinate a plan of care designed to meet your needs. Should you have any questions, feel free to call Ann at 781-999-8888. Thank you in advance for completing the questionnaire.

Sincerely,

Jane Jones, M.D.

Exhibit B. Telephone Script for Initial Assessment.

Care Manager_____   Patient Name_____
Date_____   ID_____

Purpose
- Prioritize among new Status One patients by setting an initial functional status and acuity
- Introduce the care manager
- Reinforce the separately mailed health-assessment questionnaire and care-planning visit

Instructions
- The care manager introduces him/herself by phone and gets answers to the screen. A triage nurse or another nurse or social worker may make the call as long as that person is closely aligned with the care manager.
- Make alternate arrangements if the patient is incompetent, has a language barrier, or is unavailable.

Script
The script is a general guide only. It is most important to engage the patient in conversation and provide a basis for continuing constructive contact with the care manager. Introduce yourself and ask the open-ended question, "In general how are you doing?" You will find that the patient's responses will fairly closely answer most of the questions. Explicitly ask only those questions that the patient did not talk about.

"Hello. My name is _____. I am calling from _____ ABC Medical Center/Group. Dr. _____ has asked me to call you. Did you receive a letter from your primary-care physician indicating that we would be calling? Dr. _____ would like to fully understand your situation and assure you that we are working together to meet your health needs."

(*Back-up issues to discuss if the patient brings them up:*) "There is no cost to you and everything is strictly confidential among you, me, and your health-care providers."

"It will not affect your health insurance in any way or your choice of us as your health-care providers."

"Do you have five minutes to speak with me?" (*If not, set up a time for a call and reinforce the need to fill out the mailed health-assessment questionnaire.*)

1. In general, how are you doing? (*Let the patient talk, noting answers that most closely correspond to these questions. Ask only the questions that have not already been talked about.*)

2. In the last three months, how has your health been?
   ____ Declining   ____ About the same   ____ Improving/good
   If getting worse, why? _____
   _____

3. In the past three months, have you used any of these?
   ____ Home-care/visiting nurses or aides   ____ Kidney dialysis
   ____ Ambulance   ____ Oxygen at home
   ____ Emergency room   ____ Hospital
   ____ Nursing home or rehabilitation facility?

4. How many different prescriptions or medications are you taking?
   ____ (*write the number*)
   What are they for?_____
   _____

5. Are you as active as you would like to be?   ____ Yes   ____ No
   If no, please tell me about it._____
   _____
   _____

6. Do you have concerns about your health?   ____ Yes   ____ No
   If yes, please tell me about them._____
   _____
   _____

7. Are you having problems getting the support and care you need?
   ____ Yes   ____ No
   If yes, please explain them._____
   _____
   _____

8. **Considering everything, how would you rate your health? Use a 1 to 5 scale, where 1 is poor and 5 is excellent.**

____Poor (1)   ____Fair (2)   ____Good (3)

____Very good (4)   ____Excellent (5)

"Thank you. This gets us started. Please fill out and return the more detailed health-assessment questionnaire." (*If it has not been received, confirm the address. If a home assessment is needed, introduce the idea and need.*)

"It's important that we (or you and the care manager) **meet and discuss what we can do, working together, to best address your health. When can you come in to meet me?"** (*Set up a time. Address any transportation barriers. If not ambulatory or incompetent, set up an in-home assessment.*)

Assigning an initial functional status

Use Question 8 to score the functional status.

Answer to Q 8	Functional Status #
Poor	1
Fair	2
Good	3
Very good	4
Excellent	5

Acuity

Using everything you know about the patient so far, *enter your judgment* of how soon the patient is likely to need hospitalization and/or high-acuity health care.

Hospitalization	Acuity Level
Next 1 to 3 months	1
Next 3 to 6 months	2
Next 6 to 12 months	3
1 to 2 years	4
Beyond 2 years	5
Deceased, left plan, or inappropriate	"X"

Exhibit C. Consultant Directory To Be Completed by the Lead Team, with Partial List of Topics.

Advice Topic	Expert(s)	E-Mail	Phone
AIDS			
Alcohol/substance abuse			
ALS			
Alternative therapies			
Alzheimer's			
Anticoagulants			
Asthma			
Benefits			
Blindness			
Burns			
Catastrophic care			

Exhibit D. Role Description for Consultants.

The role of the expert is to provide advice in a timely way to care managers for the purpose of developing and carrying out health action plans for Status One patients. Experts enhance the care-planning process by enabling care managers to access their knowledge of and experience with specific topics. Care managers will provide brief descriptions of their specific issues with Status One patients. Experts will provide brief but sufficient responses to these questions.

Experts are expected to:
- Check e-mail and voice mail at least daily
- Acknowledge requests for advice within twenty-four hours
- Answer most questions within twenty-four hours or indicate when a full response will be provided
- Respect the role and capabilities of care managers; understand that no question is a "dumb" question

Exhibit E. Sample Letter to New Consultant.

March 1, 2001

Consultant
ABS Health System
123 Main Street
Somewhere, USA 63108

Subject: Your Role as Consultant to Status One Patient Care Managers

Dear [name]:

You have been identified as an expert in [describe field] within the ABC Health System. The purpose of this letter is to ask for your help as a consultant to our small group of case managers who are working on a new medical management initiative.

ABC Health System is now providing medical management services to our medical centers and groups for their managed-care population. Because we are fully at risk for this population, we are diligently working to support our providers in delivering the most appropriate care while effectively managing the medical costs of this group.

We are currently implementing a new initiative to identify prospectively those of our members most likely to require high-cost care in the next twelve months. Our case managers use the technology and approach of a commercially available model in working with our physicians to proactively manage the care of these patients. These case managers assess each patient's current situation and design individualized care plans with the patient and primary-care physician in order to address the patient's medical and psychosocial needs.

As a Status One consultant, you would not be expected to have any direct contact with the patients but rather would be expected to respond to brief, targeted questions posed by the case managers as they design custom care plans for these complicated patients. The case managers will communicate with you by fax, voice mail, or e-mail in accordance with your preference. Because the case managers want to work with patients quickly and proactively, we ask that you answer their questions within twenty-four to forty-eight hours whenever possible.

Based on past experience, the volume of consultant requests for any individual is minimal, at most a few per month. I will call you in the next week to discuss your participation and your preference for how the case managers should communicate with you. In the meantime, if you have any questions, please feel free to call me at 333-4444.

Sincerely,

John Smith, M.D.
cc: Medical Director

Exhibit F. Consultant Communication Form.

Consultant's name: _____

Area of expertise: _____

Consultant's address: _____

_____

_____

Consultant's phone no.: _____

Fax no.: _____

E-mail address: _____

Preferred communication medium (check one):

_____ fax

_____ e-mail

_____ intranet

_____ voice mail

Exhibit G. Form for Identifying Possible Health Actions for a Status One Patient.

Priority	Aims	Health Actions	Response
	Coordination of medical care		
	Self-reliance		
	Daily activity and fitness		
	Interdependence with family and friends		
	Mental challenge		
	Community involvement and purpose		

Patient _____

Care Manager _____

Index

118–119, 123, 124; registries and, 40–51, 67–68; sorting methods for, 185–189; Status One approach to, versus other approaches, 123, 125; utilization rates for, 119–120, 123, 124. *See also* Predictive models; Registries; Registry, Status One; Segmentation

"Identified proactively": program design implications of, 13; Status One characteristic of, 12, 13, 23

"Ill" population segment, 21–22, 27–28

Immunization rate improvement initiative, 171

Immunological disease registries, 44

In vitro fertilization, 202

Incentives, 194–195, 205; in fee-for-service, 201; strategy of, 10–11

Incidence: concept of, 176–177; measures of, 178; prevalence and, 177–179

Inclusion criteria, in case versus care management, 129

Incompetent patients, initial contact with, 71, 72

Incremental medical management strategy, 149–150, 209–210

Independent practice associations (IPAs): clinical leadership in, 55; health maintenance organization, 197; population-segmentation methodologies of, 116; quality improvement initiatives of, 170–171; utilization rounds in, 61

Independent variable: defined, 185; in multiple regression, 185–187

Indicators, leading and lagging, 36, 39–41; disease registries and, 43–44

Infectious disease registries, 44

Information, 29–51; expert judgment and advice, 50; future research agenda for, 155–156; reference, 50; types of, 50. *See also* Data; Registries

Information technology (IT): for automation of medical records, 51;

best practices of, 211; for data integration, 29–35, 47–48; expert system, 35–36, 37–38; future research agenda on, 155–156; lead team's responsibilities for, 59; needed for population health management, 7–8, 29–30, 50. *See also* Data; Internet; Intranets; Registries

Initial contact, 71–72; exceptional situations encountered in, 71–72; telephone script for, 222

Initial visit, collaborative care planning in, 92–93

Innovations, and health care costs, 202

Inpatient days rating, 23

Inpatient severity-adjusters, 36

Inspection, quality by, 164–165

Insulin, 40, 120, 146, 147

Insurance switching, 99–100

Integrated delivery systems (IDSs): information strategies and, 29–30; predictive models used in, compared, 122–125. *See also* Risk-bearing delivery systems

Interdependence with family and friends, 88, 90

International Classification of Diseases, 9th Ed. (ICD9), 119, 120, 187–188

International Classification of Diseases (ICD) codes, 39

Internet: automated medical record and, 51; care planning resources on, 92; future research agenda of, 156; information strategies and, 29

Intestinal obstruction, 169

Intranets, 7, 8, 211; care management software for, 57, 74, 91; consultations and, 91–92; registry updates and, 48

Introductory mailing, 70–71, 223–224

Involvement, patient. *See* Patient involvement

Ishikawa charts, 166

Ishikawa, K., 159

Islands of data, 30–32